R.E.

It is widely
high blood pressure is
inspite of this knowl
worse, misunderstood.

At the heart of high blood pressure is a vicious circle: high blood pressure is a precursor of many health problems, and is in turn, produced by certain diseases.

In this easy-to-understand book, Dr Krishan Gupta explains how blood pressure is regulated by our body, why it sometimes goes out of control and what to do to maintain a healthy blood pressure. Within these pages you will find practical, everyday advice to manage blood pressure better, and to help yourself or your loved ones to lead a normal active life.

The Author

Dr. Krishan Gupta is an international authority in Internal Medicine and Geriatrics. His conviction that people should possess a working knowledge and an intelligent understanding of modern day diseases has been the motivating factor behind his authorship of numerous books, medical articles and book chapters. Although he is concerned with the recovery of health, he places equal importance on the prevention of disease. The question-answer style that he frequently adopts provides the reader with answer to doubts or questions often left unaswered by doctors.

A National and University Merit List Scholarship holder, Dr. Gupta completed his MBBS from Punjab University. He held prestigious appointments in the UK, including that of consultant physician in England. He is a currently a Professor of Medicine at the New York Medical College and a fellow of the Royal College of Physicians (UK), American College of Physician, New York Academy of Medicine and the Gerontological Society of America. During his interactions and travels in India, UK, USA and to other parts of the world, Dr. Gupta has become well-versed with the specific needs and medical problems faced by different communities and societies.

High Blood Pressure

Causes, Prevention and Treatment

Dr Krishan Gupta
MD, FRCP, FACP
Professor of Medicine
New York Medical College, USA

Orient Paperbacks
DELHI | MUMBAI | HYDERABAD

Disclaimer

The information included in this book is general in nature and for reference and guidance only. It is not a substitute for medical advice and the readers are urged to consult their doctor before taking decisions which are medical in nature.

Most drugs mentioned in the book are available in Asia and the Indian subcontinent. The brand names under which these are sold may vary from country to country.

Generic names are given in italics and brand names in capitals.

www.orientpaperbacks.com

ISBN : 978-81-222-0421-6

1st Published 2007
3rd Printing 2012

High Blood Pressure: Causes, Prevention & Treatment

Cover Design by Vision Studio

Published by
Orient Paperbacks
(A division of Vision Books Pvt. Ltd.)
5A/8 Ansari Road, New Delhi-110 002

Printed in India at
Anand Sons, Delhi-110 092

Cover Printed at
Ravindra Printing Press, Delhi-110 006

Foreword

The results of recent population studies have highlighted the enormity of the health problem posed by elevated blood pressure (hypertension). Worldwide, hypertension is found in 20 per cent of the adult population, and the condition is a major cause of premature heart disease, kidney disease and stroke. The risk of heart disease and stroke has been found to be related directly to elevated blood pressure levels.

Fortunately, the risk of elevated blood pressure has been found to be modifiable by changes in diet, exercise habits and alcohol consumption, and these interventions can also prevent high blood pressure from developing. A wide array of effective blood pressure-lowering drugs are also available to treat hypertension, with proven evidence that these medications can also reduce the risk of heart disease and stroke. Prevention and treatment of high blood pressure can only be effective if other modifiable cardiovascular risk factors are also addressed such as cigarette smoking, cholesterol elevation, obesity (increased weight) and diabetes. The challenge now is to make certain that blood pressure elevations are recognised so that appropriate lifestyle modifications and drug treatments can be instituted. At the same time, interventions need to be utilized for preventing the development of high blood pressure in susceptible individuals.

High Blood Pressure: Causes, Prevention & Treatment is an excellent source of information for anyone wanting to remain healthy. The book provides updated knowledge in an organised, readable and focussed fashion regarding the causes, diagnosis, prevention and treatment of high blood pressure. Although high blood pressure can last a lifetime, it can be controlled and the reader can play an important role in controlling it, thus the main purpose for this book. The reader will be able to understand the causes of high blood pressure, the risks of high blood pressure, how blood pressure control can save your life, and the various non-drugs and drugs available for effective blood pressure control. An informed patient who is partners with his or her healthcare provider will also achieve maximum benefit from blood pressure control interventions.

Dr. Krishan Gupta, is one of the world's leading physicians in the area of risk factor control and high blood pressure management. He is an outstanding teacher and researcher who has made many important contributions to our understanding of high blood pressure. His vast expertise in this area and his ability to communicate his knowledge effectively to readers of all backgrounds makes this book an important resource for preventing and treating a major cause of premature loss of life in our modern world.

William H. Frishman, MD, MACP
Professor and Chairman, Department of Medicine
New York Medical College, Valhalla, NY

Contents

Preface

The book is the result of my interaction with thousands of patients with high blood pressure (hypertension). Hypertension is obviously a common condition affecting millions of people around the world. Our understanding of hypertension and its treatment has changed substantially in the past twenty years. Based on strong scientific evidence, we now have learned the importance of treating high blood pressure even if it is 'mild'. Similarly, we have learned the importance of controlling hypertension in people in their later years of life. Fortunately with the availability of newer classes of medications, it has become much easier to manage this problem. It is my personal belief that a thorough understanding of a chronic condition like hypertension is essential to prevent multiple complications related to high blood pressure.

My appreciation goes to numerous patients and families with whom I have interacted over the past thirty years. More importantly, this work would not have been possible without the continuing commitment and personal interest of the publisher, Mr. Sudhir Malhotra. In addition, I am also thankful to his editorial staff for revising the text and bringing it to its present format. My wife Veena, a cardiologist, and Shalini and Sheila, my two medical daughters, also played an important role in reviewing multiple drafts and making helpful suggestions. More recently, my brother, Mr. B. K. Gupta was particularly instrumental in getting this work expedited through his meetings with the publisher in Delhi.

I sincerely hope that the readers will find this book an easy to understand guide that can help them towards the prevention and treatment of this major risk factor for heart disease, stroke and premature death.

Krishan Gupta

1

Introduction

Acute disease is an act of God, of chronic disease the patient himself is the author.

Thomas Sydenham
1624-1689

High blood pressure or hypertension is one of the most common conditions affecting the adult population in most of the Western world and is increasingly becoming common in countries such as India.

Recent scientific studies have indicated that Indians living both in India and outside have a very high prevalence of heart disease. In an American study* of coronary heart disease in people of Indian origin, Dr E. Enas, Director of the Rockford Lipid Center found that the incidence of coronary heart disease in Asian Indians in America was at least four times higher than white Americans. Not only are Indians at least 3 to 5 times

* *American Journal of Cardiology* 1992; 70: 945-949.

more at risk of developing heart attacks as compared to the local white population, but in most cases, they happen to suffer from heart attacks 5 to 10 years earlier as compared to white patients. It is a statistic that we cannot be proud of. Indians living in Fiji, Trinidad and South Africa have also been reported with higher rates of heart disease. Unfortunately, affluent Indians within India or settled abroad are almost equally at risk of developing hypertension, diabetes and heart disease.

Although precise reasons for a high rate of heart disease amongst Indians have not been fully understood, it is increasingly accepted that a large percentage fail to pay enough attention to early prevention, detection and appropriate treatment of major risk factors like hypertension and high cholesterol. Although the precise statistics are not easily available, between 20 and 25 per cent of Indian adults are estimated to suffer from hypertension.

High Blood Pressure: A Threat to Health

The importance of good control of hypertension has been confirmed by multiple studies over the past 30 years. High blood pressure, both systolic as well as diastolic, are a threat to health. Effective blood pressure control is necessary and must be done at the earliest stage. Any delay or neglect only accentuates the damage that goes with persistently high blood pressure.

There are three main organs that bear the brunt of the damage caused by uncontrolled hypertension — the heart, the brain and the kidneys. Why let these organs get damaged if appropriate control of high blood pressure can keep these healthy and in good shape?

While Western countries have shown remarkable success in reducing the rate of heart disease and stroke — the two most serious complications of uncontrolled hypertension — India still continues to have a much bigger problem with detection and proper control of hypertension. Lack of knowledge and awareness, lack of resources, poor availability of medical facilities and medications, illiteracy and poverty are some of the factors associated with poor results.

It is not that Western countries have been totally successful in bringing blood pressure under control in their entire patient population. Even with much larger resources and higher education levels, appropriate blood pressure control is being achieved in less than 30 per cent of adults in the United States. Unfortunately, no definite numbers are available for India. The best educated guess is that less than 20 per cent of Indians with hypertension have good blood pressure control. No wonder, there is an ever-increasing number of people suffering from complications of hypertension. These complications occur mainly in the form of coronary heart disease and heart attacks, congestive heart failure, strokes and kidney failure, all of which contribute to premature death.

Many of us are likely to know at least one or more individuals with hypertension, and perhaps some hypertension related complications. Personally, I am aware of at least three among family members and close friends, who died in their late forties because of failure to keep blood pressure under good control.

Facts about Blood Pressure

Let us look at some general facts about high blood pressure. Even though most adults may visit their doctor for one reason or another, between 40 and 50 per cent of those with hypertension remain undiagnosed. Of those who are diagnosed, only 50 per cent are noted to receive some treatment. And of those who do take treatment, less than 20 per cent are considered to have good blood pressure control!

A Silent Killer. Unfortunately in most cases high blood pressure produces few obvious or visible symptoms, and therefore, doctors and scientists call it a silent killer. Even today thousands of people with high blood pressure continue to remain undetected until they are rushed to the hospital with some serious, and often, life-threatening complications associated with untreated hypertension.

How do we deal with a silent killer, then? Obviously a silent killer requires a much higher degree of awareness both on the part of the patients as well as the doctors. In approximately 95 per cent of cases no obvious or clear-cut cause can be blamed for high blood pressure. This is termed as 'primary' hypertension. Many of these people have a strong family history of hypertension.

A Lifestyle Disease. Hypertension has also been termed mainly a lifestyle disease. Lack of physical exercise, smoking, obesity and high salt intake are some of the reasons that are commonly identified as contributing to high blood pressure.

A Major Risk Factor for Heart Attack. In terms of heart attacks, every individual must have some basic understanding of risk factors. Hypertension is considered to be one of the three major risk factors for heart attacks. The other two major risk factors are smoking and high cholesterol. Control of hypertension certainly remains the key for preventing premature death and improving the lifespan. It is estimated that good blood pressure control alone can achieve 20 to 25 per cent reduction of heart disease.

A Ticking Time Bomb

In recent years, India's economic and technological progress has been very impressive. Unfortunately, economic success, affluence and technical prowess do not provide immunity against lifestyle diseases like hypertension, diabetes and heart disease. If anything, by joining the rat race we only increase the risk of these 'Western' diseases.

In many ways, this is what happened in countries like England and the United States. However, as a policy, these countries now spend millions of dollars to increase awareness about the risks associated with high blood pressure. The Indian scene is somewhat different. A high percentage of Indians, including many with college degrees, still fail to understand the risk and dangers of hypertension and other lifestyle diseases. Untreated hypertension is, indeed, a ticking time bomb waiting to explode. The time to act is now.

It is no secret that the average Indian considers himself sick only if he becomes so sick and disabled that he is unable to take care of his daily routine. High blood pressure is not often regarded as a condition to be treated and many adults don't even know their blood pressure readings.

Remember, that only strict blood pressure control can save you from the dreadful complications of hypertension. Unless you are prepared to take charge of your health, high blood pressure can lead to serious complications and even premature death. Although we do not yet have a complete cure for hypertension, but with necessary lifestyle changes and some pills taken once or twice a day, blood pressure can be safely brought under complete control.

Advances in Modern Medicine

While the precise cause of high blood pressure still remains elusive, modern medicine has made significant advances in making several classes of medications available for hypertension control. Starting from the development of diuretics in the 1950s, we now have beta blockers, alpha blockers, calcium channel blockers, ACE inhibitors, etc., that are quite potent and effective in controlling hypertension.

In recent years, medical scientists have also gained better knowledge and understanding regarding the role of combination therapy (taking two or three different drugs) for the control of hypertension. Based on the studies of the benefits of hypertension therapy, hypertension treatment guidelines continue to be revised periodically. Most of these guidelines have come from the Joint National Committee on Detection, Evaluation and Treatment of High Blood Pressure in the United States. For example, we know that although the general goal of treatment must be to lower the blood pressure below 140/90 in all adults, in people with diabetes mellitus or kidney failure, blood pressure must be lowered to below 130/80. While further research remains necessary, what we already know must be practised diligently.

I hope that with the information available in this book, readers will find it easier to understand the problems and complications of hypertension and do everything possible to maintain and bring their blood pressure under control.

This book is intended not only for those who suffer from hypertension, but also for millions of those adults who are at a significant risk of developing hypertension as they enter middle and late age. With appropriate steps and a clear understanding of risk factors, the majority of you, I hope, will be able to prevent hypertension.

The message in this book is simple and clear. You must know your blood pressure. If it is high (more than 140/90 mmHg), then discuss the treatment with your doctor. There is no other solution. There are no shortcuts or magic answers. Fortunately, the treatment of hypertension is easy, effective and achievable, if you take charge of your health.

2

What is Blood Pressure?

Disease is very old, and nothing about it has changed. It is we who change, as we learn to recognise what was formerly imperceptible.

Jean Martin Charcot

Blood pressure is force of the blood against the walls of the blood vessels — the arterties and veins in the body. Without this pressure, blood would not be able to circulate in the body. There are many thousands of kilometers of these blood vessels, which are the channels or the pipes through which blood travels to all organs of the body. The heart is the principle pumping station that forces the blood through the blood vessels.

The Cardiovascular System

The cardiovascular system consists of the heart and the two main networks of blood vessels — the systemic circulation network, which supplies blood to all parts of

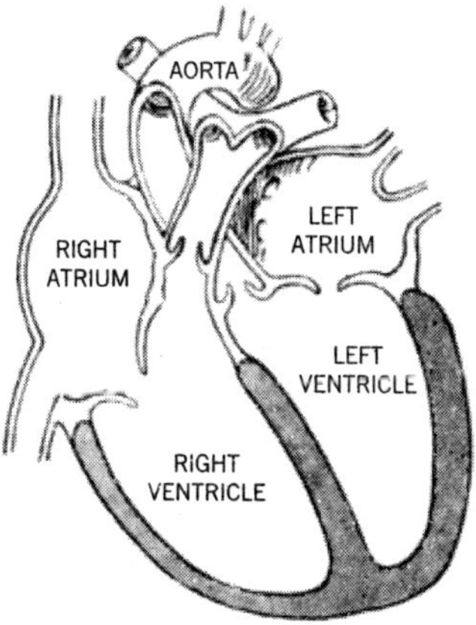

The Heart

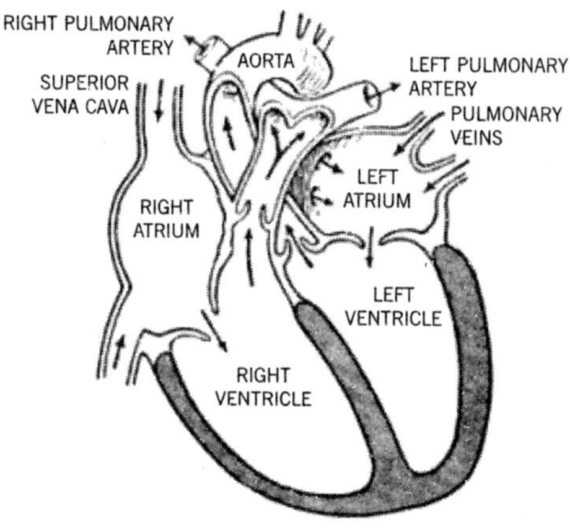

Flow of Blood through the Heart

the body except the lungs, and the pulmonary circulation which transports blood between the heart and the lungs.

The cardiovascular system circulates the blood around the body, which carries or transports nutrients and oxygen to the tissues, and also removes the waste products.

The Heart. The heart is an extraordinary organ. It is a pear-shaped muscular pump which drives blood to all parts of the body. Located in the centre of the chest, slightly inclined towards the left, it has four main chambers, two above and two below. The two upper chambers of the heart are thin walled and called atrium; the two bottom chambers with thick muscular walls are called ventricles.

The large pipe coming out of the heart into which blood is pumped is called aorta.

Arteries and Arterioles. The aorta gives rise to many arteries that are responsible for transporting blood to different organs. Typically the walls of the arteries have three different layers. The innermost layer is called the *intima*, the middle layer is called the *media* and the outermost layer is known as the *adventitia*. The contraction or relaxation of the middle muscular layer controls the blood flow in the arteries.

Amazing!

- The heart beats approximately 70 to 80 times every minute and 100,000 times per day.
- It pumps about 40,000 litres of blood per day.
- There are approximately 60,000 kilometers of blood vessels in your body.

Arteries divide into smaller pipes called arterioles. There are millions of arterioles in the body. Arterioles are further divided into still smaller blood vessels called capillaries. Pure blood releases its oxygen from these capillaries to the tissues and cells of the body. The pure or oxygenated blood, after giving up its oxygen, becomes impure by taking carbon dioxide from the cells and the tissues. The impure or deoxygenated blood is brought back to the heart through the veins. The veins empty in the right side of the heart which pumps the blood to the lungs for purification (oxygenation). Oxygenated or pure blood from the left side of the heart is, once again, pushed into the aorta with each heart beat.

The above cycle, as you can imagine, goes on at all times even when you are asleep. Several complex mechanisms are responsible for maintaining the blood pressure and blood supply to all parts of the body. Some of these, including the endocrine, nervous system, and kidneys play a major role in the maintenance of blood pressure.

Blood Pressure Maintenance

Blood pressure maintenance is a complex mechanism. In healthy individuals, there are several mechanisms that operate to keep the blood pressure within normal range. At least five different organs play an important role in this homeostasis:

1. Central nervous system — operates through changes in the sympathetic nervous system.

2. Heart — regulates the blood pressure through changes in cardiac output and heart rate.

3. Kidneys — influence blood pressure control through sodium and water absorption.

4. Adrenal glands — control blood pressure through hormonal (adrenalin) secretion.

5. Arteries and arterioles — in medical terms, these vessels constitute the vascular bed and maintain blood pressure through regulation of peripheral resistance.

The blood pressure is equal to the product of cardiac output and total peripheral resistance. In the treatment of hypertension, different drugs have different modes of actions. Since the mechanisms of action are different, it is now becoming a common practice to use two or more drugs to control high blood pressure.

Know your Blood Pressure

It is very important for everyone to know his or her own blood pressure readings. Unfortunately, many adults are simply not interested in knowing whether their blood pressure is in the normal range or not. A survey by the National Council on the Ageing in the United States, found that nearly 50 per cent of people over the age of 50 had no idea about their blood pressure readings. I'm sure you probably know at least a few such people in your family or among friends who have never bothered to check their blood pressure. Do wake up and try to find out your blood pressure numbers because, if both of your blood pressure readings are over 140/90 mmHg, you can do something about it. Hypertension is a deadly disease, but you can certainly save yourself from all the complications of high blood pressure if only you know the numbers!

3

How Blood Pressure is Measured

Everything is good when it leaves the Creator's hands; everything degenerates in the hands of man.

Jean Jacques Rousseau

When doctor takes your blood pressure, he uses an instrument known as a sphygmomanometer. It consists of an inflatable arm cuff attached to an air pump and a column of mercury or a pressure gauge. As some of you may have experienced, the rubber cuff is put around the upper arm and inflated to the point tight enough to temporarily stop the blood from passing through the brachial artery (the artery in the front of the elbow). The stethoscope is kept over the brachial artery and the doctor gradually lets the air out from the cuff. Once the pressure in the rubber cuff starts dropping, a sound becomes audible through the stethoscope and the number on the mercury column at this point becomes your systolic blood pressure (the upper number). Gradually the sound disappears altogether as the pressure is released from the cuff. At that point the sound in the stethoscope disappears and the doctor notes the number on the pressure gauge. This reading becomes your diastolic blood pressure (lower number). Although the systolic blood pressure can be measured by palpation (by fingers) or by auscultation (by stethoscope), the diastolic blood pressure can only be measured by auscultation with a stethoscope.

Systolic and Diastolic Pressure

Blood pressure is always discussed with two different numbers. The upper number is the systolic blood pressure and the lower readings are referred to as diastolic blood pressure.

Systolic Pressure. When the large pumping chamber of the heart i.e. the left ventricle contracts, a jet of blood is forced into the large arteries. The blood flows through the arteries as a 'pulse' and this causes an increase in the blood pressure already in the artery. This momentary increase in pressure is called the systolic pressure or systole.

Diastolic Pressure . The heart rests between each beat so as to gather its energy and work efficiently for a long time. Therefore after the ventricles contract, they rest for a short time while blood flows into them from the auricles. During this resting period the pressure of blood is the lowest in the arteries and this pressure is called the diastolic pressure or the diastole.

Pulse Pressure: The difference between the systolic and diastolic pressure i.e. between the high and the low is known as the pulse pressure. For example, in a person

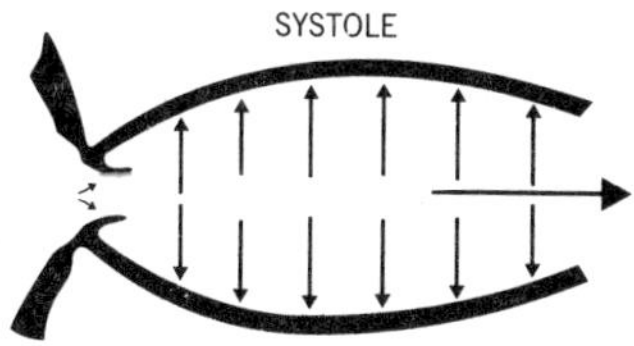

Showing expansion during cardiac systole blood flow

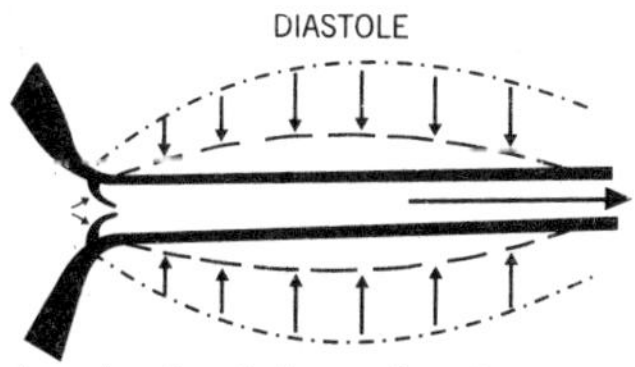

Showing relaxation during cardiac diastole blood flow

Elasticity of Walls of the Aorta

with a blood pressure of 120/80, the pulse pressure is 40 mmHg (systolic 120 - diastolic of 80 = 40 mmHg). (See also Chapter 5.)

The two numbers, systolic and diastolic, constitute the blood pressure reading in millimeters of mercury (mmHg). For example, if blood pressure is 120/80 mmHg, it simply means that you have a systolic blood pressure of 120 mmHg and a diastolic blood pressure of 80 mmHg. Initially some may find the two terms, systolic and diastolic, somewhat confusing. However, for anyone interested in maintaining a healthy blood pressure, it is strongly advised that they become familiar with these terms. Some people continue to use the terms as upper and lower blood pressure numbers, which is also fine. It is important to remember that blood pressure is never a single number. It is always given in two different numbers, systolic or the upper blood pressure reading and diastolic or the lower blood pressure reading.

Although in the past diastolic blood pressure readings were considered to be most important, in recent years we have learned to recognise the increasing role of systolic blood pressure readings.

In the Joint National Committee's sixth report, the three stages of hypertension have been based both on *systolic* as well as *diastolic* readings. Based on this classification, it is important to understand that you do not have to have both *systolic* as well as diastolic readings to be high to fall into a specific category of hypertension. Any of the readings, systolic or diastolic or both may make you join one of the three stages of hypertension.

Types of Measuring Instruments

Four different types of blood pressure instruments, or manometers, are currently available. These are:

1. *Aneroid.* These manometers utilise air pressure for measurement of blood pressure. They are usually less reliable and have a somewhat higher degree of inaccuracy.

2. *Mercury.* These manometers are most commonly used in doctors' offices. They are regarded as being more accurate and reliable than the aneroid type.

3. *Electronic.* The accuracy of electronic manometers is only comparable to the aneroid type of manometers. Since mercury manometers are considered to be more reliable, the accuracy of the electronic manometers must be checked periodically by comparison with mercury manometers.

4. *Finger recording devices.* In recent years, these fancy devices have been introduced in the market. However, they are not very reliable and tend to show a wide variability in blood pressure readings.

Ambulatory Recording

In recent years improved blood pressure measurement techniques have been developed. Ambulatory recordings is one such technique. With the ambulatory blood pressure recording system, blood pressure can be safely recorded continuously for a period of 24 hours.

Ambulatory devices are small blood pressure machines attached to the body which can record blood pressure both during the day as well as at night. These are fairly lightweight, portable and noninvasive machines and do not interfere with daily routine activities. Blood pressure readings are recorded every 15 to 30 minutes during the day and every 30 to 60 minutes at nighttime enabling a better assessment and treatment of blood pressure. However, as yet only specialised medical centres are involved in the use of these rather sophisticated machines. From the computer printout of multiple readings, the doctor is able to determine the average blood pressure both during the day as well as at night. Although some experts have argued that blood pressure readings performed over a period of 6 to 12 hours are sufficient, 24-hour monitoring is considered to be better.

Role of Ambulatory Blood Pressure Monitoring. In recent years, many hypertension experts (hypertensionologists) have argued that routine office visits by people with suspected or established hypertension are not very helpful and, therefore, to get a true picture of blood pressure, it must be monitored more accurately at different times.

What is the message? The simple conclusion is that ambulatory monitoring has a significant role in the diagnosis and management of hypertension, yet this type of testing is not needed for everyone. Depending on the total clinical picture, the doctor may decide when ambulatory monitoring is required.

Clearly, with the limited use and availability of ambulatory blood pressure machines, they are considered useful only for certain specific situations. The US Joint National Committee on Hypertension has specifically defined the role of ambulatory monitoring in their 6th report (1997) as well as 7th report (2004) for the following three situations:

1. *White coat hypertension.* If blood pressure is found to be too high in the doctor's office, ambulatory monitoring can be an indispensable tool. It obviates the common problem of white coat hypertension. It has been shown through scientific studies that ambulatory recordings are more closely correlated to complications of hypertension than readings in doctor's clinic (see chapter 5).

2. *Resistant hypertension.* If despite taking treatment, blood pressure remains high and the doctor wants to know more about blood pressure readings at different times of the day, ambulatory monitoring can play a significant role in assessing the effects of different drugs used for the control of hypertension (see chapter 7).

3. *Episodic hypertension.* Ambulatory monitoring can be utilised to confirm the diagnosis of hypertension in people with borderline hypertension and to resolve the

disparity between blood pressure readings at home and at doctor's office.

Research studies have clearly shown that ambulatory monitoring is superior in predicting and assessing the problem of left ventricular hypertrophy (see chapter 13). This enlargement of the left ventricle is a complication of untreated or poorly controlled hypertension. Dr. Guiseppe Mancia and his colleagues from Universita di Milano published the result of their study in 1997 in the journal *Circulation*. They noted from their study that both daytime and nighttime ambulatory readings correlated more closely with left ventricular mass index as compared to readings in doctors' offices.

The ambulatory monitoring system clearly has the following three distinct advantages:

1. It is more reliable than office blood pressure measurements.

2. It has less variability.

3. It has better correlation with target organ damage associated with hypertension.

Despite the above benefits, most hypertension experts do not consider ambulatory monitoring as a part of routine evaluation and treatment of hypertension. Ambulatory monitoring is certainly associated with discomfort, inconvenience and disturbed sleep. The high cost of the procedure, lack of definition for normal and abnormal blood pressure parameters, and the need for further studies are some of the reasons why ambulatory monitoring has not yet been accepted as a routine procedure.

How often should Blood Pressure be Measured

Should your blood pressure be measured every time you visit your doctor's office? It is argued that vital signs, including blood pressure, pulse, temperature and respiration, must be recorded in your medical chart every time you are seen by a doctor. The US Preventive Service Task Force and the American College of Physicians have suggested that all healthy adults should have their blood pressure checked every 1 to 2 years. Since hypertension is a major medical problem, and in most cases it does not cause any significant symptoms, I would suggest that you have your blood pressure checked at least once a year.

Guidelines for Blood Pressure Measurement

The following rules regarding blood pressure measurements must be kept in mind:

1. You must rest for a few minutes (5 to 10 minutes) before having your blood pressure checked.

2. Blood pressure may be taken lying down or sitting up.

3. The arm must be supported and positioned at the level of the heart. If the blood pressure is taken on a hanging arm, it may be found to be falsely high by 5 to 8 mmHg.

4. If one half of the body has been affected by a stroke (paralysis), blood pressure should be taken in the stronger arm. Blood pressure readings taken in the paralysed arm are not considered to be completely reliable.

5. The cuff size of the sphygmomanometer (blood pressure machine) must be of the desirable size. If the size

of the cuff is too small, it may give falsely high blood pressure readings.

The best sizes are: 12×26cm size for normal adults, 12×40cm size for obese people, 12×18cm size for children.

6. Do not have blood pressure checked if caffeine (coffee, tea) or alcohol has been taken or tobacco smoked in the last 1 to 2 hours.

7. If blood pressure is being checked the first time, it should be checked in both arms. If the blood pressure is higher in one arm, use this arm for all future blood pressure readings. Between 5 to 10 per cent of people may have some degree of obstruction to the subclavian artery (the artery going from the neck to the arm). This obstruction is likely to give a lower reading on the affected side.

8. Have blood pressure readings taken at least 2 to 3 times. Each reading may be taken at an interval of a few minutes.

9. For someone on medication for hypertension, blood pressure must be checked in a standing position as well. If there is a significant drop of blood pressure upon standing (more than 20 mmHg), then the person is considered to have postural hypotension. Postural hypotension is far more common in the older population and may result in dizziness, syncope (temporary loss of consciousness) and falls. Your doctor may need to reduce or change your blood pressure medications if you are found to have postural hypotension.

4

Normal and High Blood Pressure

When it comes to your health, I recommend frequent doses of that rare commodity — common sense.

Wincent Askey
1960

Generally speaking any adult with a blood pressure reading consistently higher than 140/90 mmHg is said to have high blood pressure or is classified as hypertensive. However, the definition and classification of hypertension has been evolving in recent years. Several of the commonly used terms like mild, moderate and severe hypertension have now been completely replaced with newer classification and terminology. For a better understanding of hypertension, it is important that you understand and acquire a working knowledge of the currently used terms.

The 7th Report of US Joint National Committee (JNC) on Detection, Evaluation and Treatment of High Blood Pressure has classified hypertension in two different stages. This classification applies to all adults over the age of 18.

Classification of High Blood Pressure

	Systolic	*Diastolic*
Optimal	< 120	< 80
Normal	< 130	< 85
High-Normal	130-139	85-89
Hypertension:		
Stage 1	140-159	90 99
Stage 2	> 160	> 100

JNC Blood Pressure Classification, 7th Report, 2004.

Based on your blood pressure readings, both the doctor and you can determine if blood pressure is normal or above normal. If you are noted to have high blood pressure, it is important to know whether it is stage 1 or 2 of hypertension.

It is important to remember that if systolic blood pressure falls under stage 1 (140 to 159) but diastolic is in the stage 2 category (100 to 109), then overall blood pressure is considered to belong to the higher category, i.e. stage 2. It is noteworthy that until the early 1990s all classification of hypertension was based on diastolic blood pressure readings only.

Furthermore, this classification applies to the period when people are not on any antihypertensive medications. Why? Because for anyone already taking medications to control hypertension, would be expected to have a blood pressure of less than 140/90.

Optimal Blood Pressure

The 7th Joint National Committee of US in its report has

made it clear that the optimal and ideal blood pressure is less than 120 mmHg systolic and less than 80 mmHg.

Normal Blood Pressure

The Committee has categorised that adults with systolic blood pressures of less than 130 and diastolic blood pressures of less than 85 have normal blood pressures. Within a normal range, there is a wide varicty of people with different blood pressure readings. Children commonly have systolic blood pressure readings of 70 to 90 mmHg and diastolic blood pressure in the range of 40 to 50 mmHg. A ten-year-old child may typically have a blood pressure of 90/50, and that is quite normal. As one grows older the blood pressure tends to rise.

Let us take the following six different persons, all with different blood pressure readings:

Normal Blood Pressure Range

Person	*Readings*
A	110/60
B	115/65
C	120/70
D	125/75
E	130/80
F	135/85

All six persons have blood pressure readings below 140/90 mmHg and therefore free from hypertension. Yet you might wonder as to which one of the six with normal blood pressure is better off in the long run.

In general, even within the normal range, the lower the blood pressure the better it is for cardiovascular health. Person A with a blood pressure reading of 110/60, for example, is at a comparatively lower risk of developing hypertension, heart attack, stroke or kidney failure as compared to person F with blood a pressure reading of 135/85.

In other words, even within the normal range, you are better off with lower normal numbers. Scientific studies have consistently confirmed that if blood pressure readings are close to the borderline blood pressure readings (around 140/90), there is a much higher risk of developing hypertension in the later years of life.

How do we know this? It is simple. Blood pressure rises with ageing and that is what would push blood pressure higher as one grows older.

In the subsequent chapters you will notice that the treatment planning has a lot to do with the degree of high blood pressure. Not all hypertensives are alike. Without strict control of blood pressure, someone with stage 2 hypertension has a far higher risk of a premature heart attack and death as compared to a person with stage 1 hypertension.

High-Normal Blood Pressure. As is clear from the classification, people with systolic of 130 to 139 and diastolic of 85 to 89 are considered to have high-normal blood pressures. The high-normal category was first created with the purpose of giving an early warning to millions of those who fell in this category. It has been widely recognised that adults with high-normal blood pressure must make significant lifestyle changes in order to prevent a further rise in the blood pressure with advancing years of life.

The High-Normal Range. What eventually happens to people if they have high-normal blood pressure has been studied by the researchers in the famous Framingham Heart Study. In order to monitor the changes in their blood pressure, people, both with normal blood pressure and high-normal blood pressure, were observed for a period of 26 years. Over this long period of observation a much higher percentage of people in the high-normal group developed definite hypertension. 54.2 per cent of men in the high-normal group eventually developed hypertension as compared to 23.6 per cent in the normal blood pressure group. In women, 60.6 per cent with high-normal blood pressure developed hypertension as compared to 36.2 per cent from the normal blood pressure group.

It is of great interest that for men weight gain over the years has been noted to correlate significantly with development of hypertension in the middle and later years of life. If the blood pressure in men is in the high-normal range, the chances of eventual hypertension are at least 2 to 3 times higher if they continue to gain significant weight (over 5 per cent of their body weight). The best bet is to control body weight if you are seriously interested in keeping your blood pressure in the normal range in the later years of life.

All stages of hypertension require medical attention and intervention. In many patients with high-normal or stage 1 hypertension, this intervention may simply be in the form of lifestyle changes.

Complications of High-Normal Blood Pressure. What should you do if you happen to have high-normal blood pressure? Is it really dangerous? The answer is yes. People with high-normal blood pressure are certainly at a greater risk of developing coronary heart disease.

The expert panel from US Joint National Committee strongly argued that the doctors must advise their patients to take appropriate steps for lifestyle changes if they have high-normal blood pressure. Most people with high-normal blood pressure can successfully reduce their blood pressure with simple lifestyle changes, including salt restriction, limiting alcohol intake, regular aerobic exercise, cessation of smoking and weight loss. If despite lifestyle changes, blood pressure fails to come down to the normal range, you may have no choice but to take one or more medications to lower the blood pressure.

Why did the JNC change the Classification?

Before the US Joint National Committee issued the current classification of blood pressure, blood pressure was labelled in terms of mild, moderate or severe hypertension. These old terms have now been abandoned. Most modern scientific textbooks of medicine emphasise that doctors stop using the old terminology and treat all patients according to the new system.

This committee of world-renowned experts emphasised that since the traditional terms simply failed to convey the seriousness of the consequences of hypertension, it would be preferable to drop terms like mild and moderate altogether.

The term mild hypertension, was deleted for very good reasons. A number of studies over the last few years have confirmed that even a mild rise of blood pressure is associated with high risk of complications of hypertension including heart attack, stroke and kidney failure. Therefore, it was decided to stay away from the term 'mild' hypertension.

In the past, when people were informed that they only had mild hypertension, they simply failed to take it seriously. As a result of this misconception, in the absence of any significant symptoms, the vast majority with mild hypertension remained untreated. Little did they understand that even a rise of 10 to 15 mmHg of blood pressure could seriously increase their risk of heart disease, stroke and kidney failure. In many ways, the medical community itself became fully aware of the complications of hypertension only in the late 1980s and 1990s. The message that the higher the blood pressure, the greater the risk of dying from complications is now no longer controversial.

So what does this mean for you? Once you know what your blood pressure readings are, you should easily be able to know your own stage of hypertension. Knowing your degree or stage of hypertension is an essential part of plan for treatment. All stages of hypertension require appropriate medical advice and treatment. Most patients with the so-called 'mild' hypertension would fall in stage 1 or stage 2 of hypertension under the new classification. With the debate conclusively settled, all patients require complete assessment and early treatment. There is simply no excuse to ignore stage 1 or stage 2 hypertension.

In any case, visiting your doctor and seeking the appropriate help and advice is your best choice.

Normal Blood Pressure Changes

The blood pressure does not stay uniform at all times. If you were to have your blood pressure checked on different occasions, either on the same day or on different days, chances are that you would not get the same readings.

Physical and emotional changes are associated with a change in blood pressure readings. For example, during sleep, the blood pressure is lower as compared to the early morning hours when you are up and about. The size of the arm cuff and the position of the arm during blood pressure recording may also matter. Let us, therefore, look into some of these seemingly simple factors that are otherwise important in the proper recording of blood pressure.

Daily Blood Pressure Changes

Your blood pressure is usually somewhat higher in the morning hours. It has been noted that heart attacks occur at least three times more commonly in the morning hours than in the evening.

In a major scientific study, Thrombolysis in Myocardial Infarction Phase II Study (TIMI II Trial)[1], it was noted that heart attacks happened 34 per cent more times between the hours of 6 am and 12 noon as compared to evening hours. Holtor Monitor (a device that records the heart beat for a prolonged period) studies have also indicated that temporary and transient myocardial ischemic (reduced blood supply to the heart muscle) episodes occur more commonly in the first 4 to 6 hours after you wake up. In one study, Marler and his colleagues clearly showed that more ischemic strokes occurred between 10 am and noon than any other 2 hour period of day.

Daily Routine and Blood Pressure. Various day-to-day activities may also influence your blood pressure, as given in the table below.

Daily Activities and Blood Pressure

Activity	*Blood Pressure*
Awake and relaxing	No change
Sleeping	Lowered 5-10 mmHg
Walking (2 miles per hr)	Rises 10-20 mmHg
Walking (3-4 miles per hr)	Rises 20-40 mmHg
Attending telephone	Rises 5-8 mmHg
Eating	Rises 3-5 mmHg
Reading	Rises 1-3 mmHg
Talking	Rises 5-7 mmHg
Sleep deprivation	Rises 5-7 mmHg
Business meeting	Rises 10-20 mmHg

The Night-time Blood Pressure. At night, when you are asleep, blood pressure tends to be lower by 5 to 10 mmHg. The drop in your blood pressure and heart rate during sleep occurs as a result of a decrease in the activity of the sympathetic nervous system; the more active the sympathetic nervous system, the higher your blood pressure. In fact, just before you wake up, towards the end of the sleeping period, the brain's sympathetic activity goes up and the blood pressure tends to rise. However, because of age related changes and somewhat poor sleep patterns, these blood pressure changes at night may not be so significant in older people. When you wake up in the morning, the alertness level rises and blood pressure goes up by 5 to 10 mmHg. During daytime, the level of physical and mental activity tends to affect blood pressure levels. Factors that may lead to a rise or fall in the blood pressure are anxiety, fear, pain, smoking, coffee intake, blood pressure cuff too narrow, and cold weather.

The Dipper and Non-Dipper Phenomena. Blood pressure starts declining during the mid-afternoon hours and continues to go down in the early part of the night almost upto 2 to 3 am. If you have a drop in blood pressure in the evening and early night hours (up to 3 am), you are considered to be a 'dipper'. For you to be classified as a dipper you must have a 5 to 10 per cent drop in blood pressure in the nighttime as compared to your daytime readings. If your blood pressure stays higher even during the nighttime, you are considered to be a 'non-dipper'.

Only in recent years, scientists and doctors have become interested in this phenomenon. Why is this so? It has been noted that non-dippers are more prone to heart attacks and strokes. So far, the dippers and non-dippers have been studied only for research purposes. As yet, doctors have not made it a part of their clinical practice to measure patients' blood pressures during the sleeping hours.

Multiple Blood Pressure Readings are needed for a Correct Diagnosis

Because of the normal changes discussed above, a single reading of blood pressure is not enough to make a diagnosis of hypertension. If you have just attended a meeting of your board of directors or have been involved in an argument, your blood pressure reading is not going to be indicative of your resting blood pressure. You may, therefore, be falsely labelled as being hypertensive if someone took your blood pressure after these stressful activities.

For example, if based on a single reading of a systolic blood pressure of 145 mmHg you were labelled as hypertensive, you may end up being started on anti-hypertensive treatment. The converse is true as well, i.e. someone who truly has mild hypertension but a single reading may show that their systolic blood pressure is below 140 mmHg.

The conclusion is that no decision should be made based solely on a single blood pressure reading. For appropriate diagnosis of hypertension, at least three different readings under restful conditions are considered to be an essential requirement.

Doctors always take at least three different readings at rest before making a diagnosis of hypertension. However, if you were started on treatment for hypertension or were told that you have hypertension based on a single blood pressure reading, perhaps you were wrongly diagnosed as having hypertension. In fact, you can help yourself by taking your own blood pressure on several different occasions in your own home under resting conditions. Home blood pressure readings can be a great help in providing a true picture about your blood pressure readings as discussed in chapter 29.

References

1. Williams, DO, Braunwald E et al; One-Year Results of the Thrombolysis in Myocardial Infarction Investigation (TIMI) Phase II Trial. *Circulation,* Vol 85, 533-542, 1992.

5

Definitions of Hypertension

Many ambitious people spend the first half of their life ruining their health to earn money and the second half spending that money to regain their health.

Bashir Qureshi, 1997
Journal of the Royal Society of Medicine

In most cases hypertension is considered to have no clear-cut underlying cause. Physicians often refer to this form of hypertension as 'primary', 'essential' or 'idiopathic' hypertension. In less than 5 per cent of cases, however, patients turn out to have a well-defined underlying cause for hypertension. These patients, therefore, are considered to have secondary hypertension (see chapter 6).

Primary or Essential Hypertension*

Primary or essential simply means a high blood pressure for which there is no known cause. The term essential

* Also called idiopathic hypertension.

hypertension was introduced many years ago and it was simply thought to result from the hardening of the arteries. This simplistic thinking is no longer accepted. Even though there are no precise known causes, a number of suspected mechanisms are believed to be responsible for this form of hypertension (see chapter 8).

Primary hypertension still remains a major form of hypertension, affecting over 90 per cent of all patients.

Borderline or Labile Hypertension

Physicians around the world still continue to use the term borderline hypertension for people whose blood pressure is noted to be somewhat higher than 140/90 mmHg on some occasions, even though the Joint National Committee for Detection, Evaluation and Treatment of High Blood Pressure in 1993 decided to completely eliminate this term.

In the past, patients with systolic readings consistently between 140 and 150 and diastolic between 90 and 94 mmHg were labelled as mildly hypertensive. If the readings were noted to be elevated on few occasions, then the physicians preferred to use the term borderline hypertension.

Another term that had also been applied to this group of patients was labile hypertension. The common factor for the use of both borderline as well as labile hypertension has been a lack of consistency in the rise of blood pressure.

In other words, the essential element of this diagnosis was the presence of higher readings only on certain occasions. But isn't it true that blood pressure varies at different times of the day? Yes, the blood pressure of a normal person is not going to be the same number at all times. However, despite this variation, blood pressure must remain within the normal range (less than 140/90) at all times. If it is a few mmHg over this limit, the term now suggested and increasingly used is stage 1 hypertension.

Is Borderline Hypertension something to Worry About?

Patients with borderline or labile hypertension have been studied by medical scientists in great detail. It has been noted that individuals with these seemingly benign abnormalities of blood pressure have some irregularities in their overall blood pressure and heart functioning in the form of increased sympathetic activity, cardiac output and rapid heart rate even at rest.

Most patients who had been labelled as borderline or labile hypertensive are noted to fall in the category of either high to normal type or stage 1 hypertension category. A person with blood pressure in the high-normal range is far more likely to develop stage 1 hypertension within a period of 10 to 15 years. Studies have also indicated that there is an increased risk of developing hypertension in later years of life for those with current blood pressure in the high-normal group.

If your doctor is still talking about borderline or labile hypertension it is best to discuss this issue and find out whether you have high to normal or stage 1 type of hypertension. It is likely that despite the use of older terms, you were still getting the right treatment for hypertension from your doctor. However for a better understanding it is best to use the currently accepted terms for hypertension and then follow the recommended treatment accordingly.

Severe, Accelerated and Malignant Hypertension

Severe and accelerated hypertension are terms that reflect a very high degree of blood pressure.

Severe Hypertension. Anyone with stage 2 hypertension with a systolic blood pressure of 180 mmHg or over, and diastolic of 110 or over, should be considered to have severe hypertension.

Accelerated Hypertension. In accelerated hypertension, the systolic blood pressure is over 180 mmHg and the diastolic is usually over 120 mmHg.

Malignant Hypertension. In malignant hypertension the systolic readings are above 200 and diastolic are between 120 and 140.

Commonly recorded readings for severe, accelerated, malignant hypertension and hypertensive encephalopathy are as below.

	Systolic BP	*Diastolic BP*
Severe	> 180	> 110
Accelerated	> 180	> 120
Malignant	> 200	120-140
Hypertensive Encephalopathy	> 200	120-140

As a result of a sustained rise of blood pressure, the vital organs of the body, including the brain, heart, kidneys and eyes, get adversely affected. With very high blood pressure readings, the evidence of end-organ damage is eventually seen in these organs. For example, someone with accelerated hypertension is commonly noted to have haemorrhages and exudates in the retina of the eye. People with malignant hypertension also have papilledema (swelling of the optic disc) along with the excessively high blood pressure readings. In malignant hypertension, there may also be signs and symptoms of kidney and heart failure. Patients with hypertensive encephalopathy typically have headaches, confusion, seizures, and eye changes of malignant hypertension.

All of the above conditions associated with grossly high blood pressure readings require urgent control and close medical supervision. Based on the situation a few days of hospitalisation may even be required. Any neglect or delay in the treatment can prove to be life-threatening. Fortunately, with a variety of currently available medications, it has become much easier to control all grades and stages of hypertension.

High Systolic Blood Pressure/Isolated Systolic Hypertension (ISH)

Several scientific reports over the past 10 years have concluded that systolic blood pressure readings may be even more important in having a closer correlation with the long-term complications of hypertension. Because many doctors were trained at a time when diastolic blood pressure was considered to be the most important blood pressure reading, they still tend to ignore the systolic readings.

There is more than sufficient scientific evidence to closely link high systolic blood pressure with a high risk of heart disease, stroke and kidney failure. In a study published in September 1999 in the British journal *Lancet*, it was pointed out that high systolic blood pressure was also a risk factor for excessive bone loss in elderly women. In their study, the researchers included 3,676 healthy women with a mean age of 73. The authors monitored the bone loss with regular bone density measurements and found that elderly women with hypertension had excessive bone loss resulting probably due to abnormal calcium metabolism and calcium loss in the urine.

Patients with high systolic blood pressure readings alone are often referred to have isolated systolic hypertension (ISH). Most of these patients tend to be elderly. The blood vessels in old age become stiffer and lose their elasticity. This loss of compliance of blood vessels is thought to result in high systolic blood pressure readings in old age.

Dr Claude J. Lenfant, the Director of the National High Blood Pressure Education Program, has called systolic hypertension a major health threat specially for older people. The old belief that 100 plus your age was an acceptable systolic blood pressure has now been found to be totally baseless and indeed very harmful. This is clearly the reason why older people should also not have a blood pressure reading of more than 140/90 mmHg according to the current hypertension classification.

A recent clinical advisory issued by the US National Heart, Lung and Blood Institute has emphasised that systolic blood pressure is more important than diastolic blood pressure for the management of hypertension in middle and old age.

Role of Pulse Pressure

In recent years, physicians and researchers have tried to understand the role of pulse pressure in cardiovascular health and disease. In one recent scientific study the American Heart Association, indicated that pulse pressure was very closely associated with long-term complications of hypertension. Although further studies are in progress, it is being widely accepted that for good blood pressure control, both systolic as well as diastolic numbers must be looked at very carefully. It has been noted that if pulse pressure remains over 50 mmHg or more, the risk of cardiac complications becomes significantly high and pulse pressure must not be allowed to be over 50 mmHg.

In a study reported in the *Journal of American College of Cardiology* in August 2000, Viola Vaccarino and her colleagues from Yale University School of Medicine decided to follow a group of 2152 older people with no evidence of heart disease. Over a period of ten years, it was calculated that with each 10 mmHg rise in pulse pressure, the heart disease risk increased by 12 per cent, heart failure risk went up by 14 per cent and the risk of death due to heart disease increased by 6 per cent.

In a research study published in the *Archives of Internal Medicine* in October 2000, Robert J. Glynn and his colleagues from Harvard Medical School reported that the highest number of people with cardiovascular deaths were noted to have the largest pulse pressure. Based on these results the study concluded that pulse pressure is the best single measure of blood pressure in predicting mortality in older people.

Pulse pressure is now believed to be the single best predictor of cardiac disease, especially in the older population.

Pseudohypertension

Pseudohypertension simply means a falsely elevated blood pressure. In pseudohypertension, the intra-arterial, or the true blood pressure, is actually normal but the cuff measurement of blood pressure reflects higher readings.

This is a problem seen mainly in older people. The elderly often have a hardening of arteries because of calcium and fat deposition in the walls of the arteries. Due to the rigidity of the arterial walls, the physician may get a falsely high reading of blood pressure.

The condition of pseudohypertension can only be safely diagnosed by a doctor. In general, all physicians must look into the issue of pseudohypertension before they start medication treatment in older patients. Older patients with no evidence of end-organ damage (normal heart, kidneys and eye findings), with high blood pressure readings are often suspected of suffering from pseudohypertension. A careful physical examination with findings of hardened calcified arteries should make the

> **Why Pulse Pressure is Important?**
>
> To know your own risk of future heart disease as you grow older, it may be wiser to focus on your pulse pressure alone. For example, a person with blood pressure readings of 170/70 (the pulse pressure of 100) has a higher long-term cardiac risk of dying from heart disease as compared to someone with blood pressure readings of 170/110 (the pulse pressure of only 60).

doctor suspicious of this diagnosis. These days ambulatory blood pressure readings are considered to be more reliable in ruling out the diagnosis of pseudohypertension.

White Coat Hypertension

It has been noted that when people visit their doctor's office, they often become nervous and anxious. Many people simply find it too difficult to relax in a doctor's office or the hospital. What are the consequences then? Their blood pressure readings are inevitably found to be high and they are often labelled as hypertensive. It has been found that blood pressure readings at home or even 24 hour ambulatory readings tend to be lower in many of the same patients who happen to have higher readings in the doctors' offices. In most cases, such patients are noted to have higher systolic blood pressure readings in the medical offices; the diastolic blood pressure readings are less commonly affected. It has been estimated that between 10 to 20 per cent of all hypertension patients may fall in this category. Since this false rise in blood pressure has been noted mostly in the medical offices and the hospitals, this phenomenon is often referred to as 'White Coat Hypertension'.

Some interesting studies have also revealed that if the blood pressure readings were taken by the nurses and not by the doctors, the 'white coat effect' is simply not there. Based on these observations, it has been suggested that office blood pressure readings are best taken by the nurses.

Can White Coat Hypertension develop into true Hypertension? Questions have often been raised regarding the precise significance of white coat hypertension. Is this a totally benign phenomenon? Does it mean that if blood pressure in doctor's office is high and readings at home are within normal range, then there is no problem? The answer is probably yes. You are not considered to have hypertension if blood pressure readings at home are repeatedly noted to be within normal range.

It has been observed that just like people with high-normal blood pressure, a significant percentage (upto thirty three percent) of people with white coat hypertension tend to develop true hypertension.

Since white coat hypertension may predispose one to develop true hypertension in later years of life, everything possible should be done to lead a healthier lifestyle and to prevent hypertension.

Despite this white coat hypertension does not require any treatment.

6

Secondary Hypertension

Diagnosis means finding the cause of a disorder, not just giving it a name.

Sydney Walker III
1996

Secondary high blood pressure refers to high blood pressure that has a known cause. The doctors are able to identify the condition or illness that triggers the blood pressure to increase. As opposed to primary high blood pressure, which can be treated but not cured, secondary high blood pressure can often be cured. Once the underlying cause is eliminated, blood pressure tends to correct itself and often return to normal.

Secondary high blood pressure occurs in less than 5 per cent of high blood pressure cases. It should be suspected:

1. If there is hypertension before the age of 30 or after the age of 60 years.

2. If blood pressure is proving to be difficult to control with the usual medications (resistant hypertension).

3. If blood pressure is too high (accelerated or malignant hypertension).

The common causes of secondary hypertension are renal, endocrine and several other diseases.

Let us look at some of these diseases in detail.

Renal Diseases

Hypertension that develops because of an underlying kidney disease is called secondary hypertension. The kidneys play an important role in the control of blood pressure. If, for some reason, the blood supply of one or both kidneys is compromised, blood pressure will almost certainly go up.

Several forms of kidney diseases have been recognised to cause hypertension. Narrowing of the arteries of the kidneys (Renal Artery Stenosis) may cause constriction of blood vessels and hypertension. While younger people may develop renovascular hypertension due to structural thickening of the renal arteries (fibromuscular dysplasia), in older people it is usually due to the generalised process of atherosclerosis.

Based on physical examination, doctor may suspect renal artery stenosis. Specialised kidney tests including ultrasound, IVP, angiography or kidney scans and captopril tests, etc. maybe required to determine the precise nature of the kidney disease. The choice of these tests is based solely on the patient's condition and the availability of procedures.

Other kidney diseases which may lead to hypertension include:

- Glomerulonephritis (inflammation of glomerular membrane, the filtering part of the kidney).

- Pyelonephritis (characterised by fever, flank pain and increased frequency of urination caused by infection in the kidneys).
- Polycystic kidney disease (caused by presence of multiple cysts in the kidney).
- Hydronephrosis (enlargement of the kidney due to obstruction in the urinary tract).

With the wide choice of drugs, including ACE inhibitors, beta blockers and calcium channel blockers, it has become easier to control blood pressure in cases of renovascular hypertension. However, in almost all of secondary hypertension, it is wise to treat the underlying condition causing the hypertension. In some cases surgical repair of the narrowed artery of the kidney is considered to be the treatment of choice. If expertise is available, angioplasty of the renal artery may also achieve similar results. In any case, once the patency of the renal arteries is restored, the blood pressure can be expected to return to normal and there should no longer be the need for antihypertensive medications.

It may not even be necessary to take blood pressure medications for the rest of your life if the hypertension was caused by a treatable kidney diseases.

Endocrine Diseases

Three of the most common conditions that require some basic understanding for our purposes are — Primary Aldosteronism (high levels of aldosterone secretion), Cushing's Syndrome and Pheochromocytoma.

Primary Aldosteronism. The adrenal gland is a small gland located near the upper end of each kidney. The outer part of the adrenal gland is known as the cortex and it secretes androgen, glucocorticoid and mineralocorticoid hormones. With a complex mechanism, these hormones control body metabolism and maintain the electrolyte balance in the body. In primary aldosteronism, the excessive production of aldosterone may cause excessive sodium and water retention and leading to hypertension. Based on the history, physical examination and blood tests (sodium, potassium levels, etc.), the doctor may suspect these conditions. The confirmation of the diagnosis invariably requires further specialised tests.

Cushing's Syndrome. In Cushing's Syndrome, excessive glucocorticoid hormones are produced. Patients with Cushing's syndrome are often obese with a round facial appearance (moon-shaped face). Once again, if suspected, the physician would need specialised tests (blood cortisol levels and CT scans of adrenal gland, etc.) to confirm the diagnosis of Cushing's syndrome. If the adrenal gland is found to have a tumour, the surgical resection of tumour is the treatment of choice.

Pheochromocytoma. In case of hypertension which is episodic and associated with pallor, nausea, headaches and palpitation then pheochromocytoma maybe suspected. A specialised blood and urine test (blood catecholamine levels, VMA excretion test) and CT scans are necessary to localise the tumour.

Hyperthyroidism. This is a comparatively common condition that may also result in hypertension. Weight loss despite an increased appetite, a rapid heart rate, excessive sweating and prominent eyeballs are some of the common features of hyperthyroidism. Simple thyroid activity test is needed to confirm diagnosis. Once diagnosed, hyperthyroidism is an easy condition to treat.

Other Causes

There may be several other reasons for high blood pressure and the doctor may want to identify that the following conditions are not the cause.

Coarctation of Aorta. A congenital heart condition that is characterized by narrowing of the aorta, the main blood vessel coming out of the left ventricle. In this condition, the blood pressure readings are typically high in the arms but low in the legs. A significant difference of blood pressure measurement in the upper and lower limbs and x-ray of the chest are sufficient for your physician to confirm this diagnosis. Surgical treatment is necessary to correct this problem.

Quadriplegia. Quadriplegia (weakness of all four limbs) commonly results from severe traumatic injury to the spinal cord. Overstimulation of the sympathetic nervous system is presumed cause of high blood pressure in these cases.

Lead Poisoning. Lead found in paints, cans and leaded petroleum can cause lead poisoning that may have adverse affects on the brain (convulsions, dementia), blood (anemia) and high blood pressure. With increasing use of lead free petrol and paint, problem of lead poisoning is on the decline.

Sleep Apnea. A condition that is characterized by disordered breathing. Snoring is the hallmark of sleep apnea and the condition is more common in obese people. High blood pressure results from low oxygen saturation of blood during the disturbed pattern of breathing in these patients. Once the diagnosis is established, sleep apnea can be successfully treated with weight loss and nasal continuous positive airway pressure (CPAP). If you suffer from snoring and have high blood pressure, you must discuss the problem with your doctor.

Contraceptive Pill

Despite low dosage preparations, oral contraceptive pills are not totally free from side effects. High blood pressure, stroke, heart attacks and breast cancer are some of the side effects of these pills. Fortunately, in most women, hypertension developing as a result of these pills is only mild and is reversible in up to 60 per cent of women if they stop taking the pills.

In recent studies, the researchers have pointed out that women taking oral contraceptive pills and hormones need close supervision and medical monitoring because of the associated risk of cardiovascular complications and hypertension.

If your blood pressure is noted to be going up, the physician may have to discontinue the use of contraceptive pills and suggest an alternative method of birth control. If the contraceptive pills must be used, the physician may decide to add an antihypertensive medication to bring your blood pressure under control. In any case, blood pressure must remain under control below 140/90 mmHg.

7

Resistant Hypertension

A person is as old as his arteries.

What if someone is taking medications and yet the blood pressure refuses to come under control?

Medically speaking, hypertension is said to be resistant only if blood pressure does not go down to normal limits despite medication. While one single drug is successful in reducing the blood pressure in 50 to 60 per cent of patients, with the use of two or more medications, the blood pressure reduction can be expected in 85 to 90 per cent of patients. Physicians often refer to patients as having resistant or refractory hypertension if the blood pressure remains high despite taking two or three different medications in the usual doses.

Questions to ask if you have Resistant Hypertension. It is not that nothing further can be done to lower blood pressure if a person happens to have resistant hypertension. Check the following to see if your blood pressure is resistant to the usual treatment:

1. Is the prescribed medications being taken sincerely?

2. Are appropriate doses of the pills being taken? If the doses are too small, you need to take appropriate action. If by mistake you took only half the dose of a blood pressure-lowering medication, your blood pressure is not likely to respond satisfactorily. Unfortunately, these innocent errors are all too common.

3. Is your lifestyle interfering with the control of blood pressure? For example, if you are going through an unusual period of stress in life, the usual doses of antihypertensive medications may not be sufficient to control blood pressure.

4. Is there too much salt in the diet? Although not everyone is salt sensitive, between 40 to 50 per cent of adults are known to be highly sensitive to salt intake. In salt sensitive people, the blood pressure goes down by 5 to 15 mmHg within a few weeks of reducing the salt intake.

5. Is too much caffeine being consumed? Excessive caffeine consumption can easily affect blood pressure. Adults taking more than four cups of coffee per day may notice that their blood pressure goes up by 5 to 10 mmHg.

6. Is there excessive alcohol intake? While one or two drinks per day are considered to provide cardiovascular protection, excessive drinking is known to raise blood pressure. If blood pressure is not responding well to the medication, it is worthwhile to reduce alcohol intake to not more than one drink per day. A better approach may be to stop drinking for a few weeks and monitor whether this helps in lowering the blood pressure to desirable levels.

7. Is some other medication being taken which possibly interferes with the control of blood pressure? Hypertension is considered to be an age-related problem. Unfortunately, several other diseases including arthritis, diabetes mellitus, obesity and heart disease are also common in the later years of life. Not surprisingly, many adults in their late 50s and 60s are forced to take one or more pills. Commonly used medications for arthritis, such as non steroidal antiflammatory agents, may cause salt and water retention and thus interfere with the control of hypertension. Even the newer agents, such as cox-2 inhibitors (Rofecoxib and Celecoxib) may also contribute to a rise in the blood pressure. So, if you think you have resistant hypertension, discuss all your current medications, including the ones that you bought over the counter (non-prescription), with your doctor.

8. Has there been excessive weight gain during the recent months? The weight gain may have happened due to a combination of factors including declining physical activity and increased calorie intake. If you have gained 5 to 10 kgs during the past 6 to 12 months, this weight gain alone could explain the difficulty in controlling your hypertension.

9. Is it possible that there maybe secondary hypertension? Between 10 to 20 per cent of patients with resistant hypertension have secondary hypertension. If your blood pressure fails to respond to a combined treatment with 2 to 3 different blood pressure pills, the question of secondary hypertension must be entertained. Depending upon the clinical examination, it is only for the doctor to rule out those secondary causes.

8

The Risk Factors

A glutton digs his grave with his teeth.

French proverb

Although tremendous amount of medical research has been carried out with thousands of studies conducted and millions of dollars spent in an effort to understand the causes of a complex disease like hypertension yet no definite cause or causes have been established. All this has however not been wasted. What is reasonably certain is that there is no one single cause in overwhelmingly majority of the cases. Most scientists believe that hypertension is due to a number of different underlying causes, the most important of which could be generic factors like heredity. Other causes also considered to predispose a person to high blood pressure are hardening of arteries, tension and stress, environment and personality, high salt diet and a tendency to overweight. We also know that the secondary causes of hypertension are responsible for approximately 3 to 5 per cent of all hypertensive cases (see chapter 6).

Heredity

It is no secret that genes have a lot to do with the medical conditions that you are likely to suffer throughout your life. These are diseases that have a strong genetic basis i.e. they run in families. Hypertension is one such disease.

The inheritance of hypertension is considered to be multifactorial. Several genetic factors are probably responsible for the development of hypertension in children of hypertensive parents.

Biological children of hypertensive parents are noted to have higher blood pressure readings in increasing numbers. There have been cases recorded of twins developing a high degree of hypertension at about the same age even though they were living in two separate cities in totally different environments. On the other hand, no correlation of blood pressure levels is noted in parents and their adopted children.

In general, if one parent has a history of hypertension, the children have approximately a 25 per cent risk of developing hypertension. With both parents having hypertension, the risk rises to up to 90 per cent.

It is important to recognise that hereditary hypertension often manifests itself when you are in your 30s or 40s. Both men and women are predisposed to develop hypertension if one or both parents had a history of hypertension.

How people with a family history of hypertension develop hypertension in their 30s and 40s still remains unclear. It is believed that environmental factors together with genetic factors are responsible for this rise in blood pressure. In other words, since a person with a strong family history of hypertension already has a genetic predisposition to developing hypertension, environmental factors such as high salt intake, low potassium intake or high alcohol consumption can precipitate the situation and make a person with high to normal blood pressure develop high blood pressure, i.e. become a true hypertensive.

Because of the genetic risk, doctor must always be informed of the family history of hypertension.

Gender

Hypertension is far more common in men than in women. The mechanisms of the development of hypertension are considered to be no different in men than in women. However, it has been noted that vascular resistance is lower in women. The overall rate and severity of complications of hypertension are noted to be much higher in men than women. While the Joint National Committee on Hypertension considers males over 55 as an identifiable risk factor, women over the age of 65 are considered to be in the same risk category. Despite these differences, hypertension must not be considered a benign disorder for women at any age.

Age

In many diseases, increasing age itself becomes a risk factor. Scientific studies have confirmed that chances of developing hypertension increase with increasing age. In other words, advancing age does pose an increasing risk developing high blood pressure.

Although not universally true, with advancing age, the systolic as well as the diastolic blood pressures tend to go up. It has been reported that while the systolic blood pressure continues to rise even after the age of 60, the diastolic blood pressure becomes stable or may even go down a little bit after the age of 60. Much of the rise in blood pressure is traced to the hardening and narrowing of the arteries. Because of the higher systolic readings in old age (with no rise in the diastolic blood pressure), many elderly people tend to have isolated systolic hypertension with wide pulse pressure (the difference between systolic and diastolic blood pressure readings). If you are one of these individuals, you need to see your doctor for appropriate management of your hypertension. Currently, the committee of experts on hypertension strongly believes that, irrespective of your age, you must not have a blood pressure reading of over 140/90. Higher blood pressure readings as part of ageing process are no longer accepted.

Stress and Personality

Psychological stress is considered to be a cause of great concern since it plays a significant role in causing many lifestyle diseases, including hypertension and heart disease. Many studies have concluded that people with high stress jobs suffer from hypertension far more frequently. People living in a close, protected environment, with a strong family support system have been noted to have less hypertension then the urban population with a less satisfactory support system. In one study researchers reported that air traffic controllers working under high stress were at least five times more likely to develop hypertension as compared to non professional pilots of the same age. The high incidence of hypertension in the Black population in the United States is also believed to occur due to high level of their anger and social stress.

People with type A personality (see page 127) usually have higher degrees of anxiety, anger, fear and stress. Therefore, it is not very surprising that adults with type A personality are more prone to hypertension and heart disease as compared to adults with type B personality.

It is no secret that anxiety, anger and depression are all your enemies. These negative qualities not only damage the cardiovascular system but also have other negative effects on the total body system.

Although a lot of stress may be related to poverty, rising prosperity does not always make people happier. It is, of course, wrong to assume that the pursuit of happiness is the same thing as the pursuit of prosperity. It has been argued that as compared to some 25 years ago, Americans are far more prosperous today, yet several surveys have confirmed that they are less happy and more stressful than ever before. In many developing countries like India, rising incomes have not resulted in higher levels of happiness and contentment. Andrew Oswald from Warwick University in England, a research expert in the area of the link between wealth and well being, has noted that wealth and human well being are not directly related at all.

The message here is very clear. Learn how to control your stress level. Those who are consistently on the run are certainly putting their health at risk and are more likely to develop hypertension and heart disease. Successful handling of stress has been shown to be very helpful in the adults.

Excessive Weight Gain and Obesity

Obesity is on the rise in almost all affluent societies around the world. In a rich country like the United States, over 50 per cent of people are known to be overweight. In India obesity is fast becoming a problem, especially in the sedentary urban population.

Dr Kanell[1] and his colleagues reported from the Framingham Heart Study that with every 5 kg of weight gain, there is a rise in systolic blood pressure of approximately 4.5 mmHg. Several epidemiological studies have established that risk of developing hypertension increases with continuing weight gain. The problem of weight gain leading to hypertension has been noted in almost all socioeconomic groups, both in men as well as in women.

Obesity is often an insidious problem that most commonly starts in the late 20s or early 30s. In an interesting study conducted at the Center for Disease Control in Atlanta, United States[2], it was noted that both for men as well as women, most weight gain took place during the ages of 35 to 44 years. The authors of the study concluded that, in general, people need to regularly monitor their body weight and keep it in check, starting at a much earlier age.

In children, with the increasing consumption of junk food and time spent watching television and with computers, video games etc the level and time spent on physical activity continues to go down. Concern regarding the rising obesity rate has therefore been expressed by many experts. Since hypertension is more prevalent in obese than in non-obese children, paediatricians and experts in adolescent medicine have urged parents not to let their children become obese. An increasingly sedentary lifestyle is perhaps the single most important reason for increasing obesity in younger adults.

Obesity not only increases the risk of developing hypertension but several other diseases as well such as diabetes mellitus, high cholesterol, coronary heart disease, strokes, osteoarthritis, falls, circulatory problems like venous thrombosis, gallstones and cancers (breast, colon, etc.)

Although the precise reasons for the development of hypertension in obesity still remain unclear, there is little doubt that putting on extra weight is almost certainly putting you at risk of developing hypertension.

A combined approach of reducing calorie intake and regular exercise is considered to be your best choice for weight reduction. A well balanced but low calorie, low fat diet can provide you with the desired result of weight loss if followed in a disciplined manner. Portion sizes must be kept smaller. Obesity is one area where prevention is much easier and better than a cure.

High Salt Diet

Although the relationship of salt intake and hypertension still remains unsettled, there is increasing scientific evidence that the risk of developing hypertension is much greater if salt intake is high. Population studies in different countries with varying amounts of salt intake have suggested that people with high salt consumption are likely to have higher blood pressure readings. Japan is a good example. Because of their high salt intake, the Japanese tend to have far more hypertension than many other nationalities. A fast lifestyle associated with packed and tinned foods with their high salt content, has only made matters worse in most of the Western world.

Not every individual has the same degree of salt sensitivity. There are of course many people who continue to take large amounts of salt and yet their blood pressure seems to be within the normal range. It is argued that approximately 50 per cent of all adults are salt sensitive, i.e. an excessive amount of salt intake is likely to cause a rise in blood pressure.

Tea and Coffee

Through its effect on different chemicals in the body (raising renin and catecholamine levels) caffeine increases your blood pressure in the same way as alcohol. One to two cups of coffee have been found to have little effect on your blood pressure. However, excessive amounts of coffee may raise your blood pressure by 3 to 10 mmHg. Since tea has less caffeine than coffee, perhaps it is a better choice than coffee as far as your cardiovascular system is concerned.

Alcohol Abuse

Alcohol has an effect on blood pressure. Within 15 to 20 minutes of taking 1 to 2 drinks of wine or whisky, your blood pressure is likely to rise between 5 to 10 mm. However, 1 to 2 drinks a day have been found to be good for your overall cardiovascular health. Since three or more drinks do cause a significant rise in blood pressure, such drinking could be considered as alcohol abuse for our working definition.

The upper limit of two drinks per day may not be suitable for everybody. Many adults, because of the pressure effects of alcohol, may have increased blood pressure even with two drinks. For such individuals, the upper limit of alcohol intake may even be one drink per day. Women in general have increased sensitivity to alcohol intake. Therefore, their limit of alcohol consumption may have to be simply one drink a day. Despite the cardiovascular benefits of alcohol, the risk of alcohol abuse remains a potential threat to health.

Smoking

Smoking has been recognised as a major risk factor for heart disease and lung cancer. But smoking also has a harmful effect on blood pressure. Smoking triggers secretion of a chemical called norepinephrine, which causes constriction of the blood vessels and in a few minutes, raises blood pressure. It is in the best interest of persons with high blood pressure to stop smoking. It not only results in better control of hypertension, but also reduces substantially the risk of heart disease. The carbon monoxide and nicotine in cigarettes are harmful to both the well-being of arteries and the regular beating of your heart.

References

1. Kannel WB, Brand N, Skinner JJ, et al. The relation of adiposity to blood pressure and development of hypertension: the Framingham Study. Ann Intern Med. 1976;67:48-49.
2. Dollemore, Doug; Raymond, Cathy; Rodale Press, Disease Free at 60-Plus: Hundreds of Life-Preserving Tips and Techniques to Defy Heart Trouble, Cancer and Stroke. *Trim Down to Trim Your Disease Risk* (Dr. David F Williamson, PhD, Centers for Disease Control and Prevention in Atlanta). Emmaus, Pennsylvania, USA, Rodale Press, 1997.

9

Medications that Cause Hypertension

He is always right who suspects that he makes mistakes.

Spanish proverb

Both newer as well as older medications can cause high blood pressure. Almost all medications have some side effects; sometimes even the apparently harmless and over-the-counter drugs may also be responsible for raising blood pressure.

Commonly available over-the-counter medications for cold, flu and weight loss have recently come to the attention of scientists for contributing to high blood pressure. In October 2000, the United States Food and Drug Administration (FDA) was asked by an expert panel of scientists to ban phenylpropanolamine (PPA), a chemical that is a common ingredient of many cold medications. Even common cough syrups containing dextromethorphan, guaifenesin and pseudoephedrine hydrochloride and appetite suppressants like Dexatrim have PPA that may raise the blood pressure and cause brain haemorrhage and strokes. The FDA has now banned the use of PPA in the United States.

Although over-the-counter or non-prescription medications are likely to have a higher margin of safety, they do have their own problems. Commonly used medications that may increase your blood pressure are:

Corticosteroids. Steroids are commonly used for allergy, asthma, eczema or inflammatory bowel disease. Because of their gluco-corticoid or mineralo-corticoid properties, steroids lead to sodium and water retention in the body and may raise blood pressure. In most cases, it is the long-term use of steroids that should become a matter of concern as far as blood pressure is concerned. Along with raising blood pressure, these drugs may also lead to congestive heart failure because of fluid retention in the body.

Monoamine Oxidase Inhibitors (MAO inhibitors). These drugs due to their sympathetic activity commonly lead to constriction of the blood vessels. Cocaine addicts often end up with high blood pressure because of excessive secretion of adrenaline from the nerve endings. Amphetamines are also responsible for stimulating the sympathetic nervous system and raising blood pressure. MAO inhibitors have been commonly used in the past for the treatment of depression and other psychiatric conditions. Occasionally, if patients on MAO inhibitors happen to consume cheese or red wine, there is possibility of a severe hypertensive crisis resulting from a chemical substance called tyramine that is found in cheese and red wine. Individuals taking MAO inhibitors, should be very careful and stay away from cheese or red wine.

Non-steroidal Anti-inflammatory Agents (NSAIDs). Arthritis and rheumatism are common problems affecting millions of adults, especially in old age. Motrin and Motrin-type drugs are freely available without a prescription. Besides stomach ulcers, fluid retention and rise in blood pressure are some of the side effects of this class of drugs. Everyone taking an NSAID must keep an eye on his/her blood pressure. Furthermore, someone already suffering from hypertension and taking NSAIDS, may find blood pressure control being affected adversely.

Medications that may raise Blood Pressure

Medications	*Commonly used for*
Ephedrine Sulfate, Pseudo-sphedrine Hydrochloride	Cold, nasal congestion, allergy
Naphazoline Hydrochloride	Eye/nose drops for decongestion
Ibuprofen and other non-steroidal agents	Analgesics for arthritis and rheumatism
Steroids	Allergy, asthma, rheumatoid arthritis, collagen diseases
MAO Inhibitors	Psychotic conditions

Erythropoetin. This is a comparatively new drug that is used for the treatment of anaemia in patients with kidney failure. Upto 30 per cent of patients taking erythropoetin are noted to have high blood pressure. Fortunately it is a rare medication and the doctor will almost certainly be aware of this problem of high blood pressure associated with erythropoeitin use.

10

Need for Control

Many look, but few see.

Maxwell M. Wintrobe
1980

The fact that high blood pressure is a major health hazard and bad for the heart has been known for many years. Anyone suffering from hypertension remains at a high risk of developing one or more complications associated with it in the next 5 to 10 years. However, it is only in recent years that the role of strict control of hypertension has received more attention than ever before.

Experts globally have been pointing out the high financial cost of treating stroke, conjestive heart failure and heart attack, the three major complications of poor blood pressure control. In the United States alone, the cost of caring for heart and stroke patients is estimated to be almost $260 billion per year. This represents over 25 per cent of the total health care cost in the United States.

Reasons for Poor Control of Blood Pressure

Despite very good evidence that blood pressure control helps in saving lives, you might wonder why so many people with hypertension remain undiagnosed or poorly controlled. This is all the more alarming considering that there are many more choices of treatment available today than 25 to 30 years ago. If in a country like USA, where health care awareness and treatment facilities are perhaps the best in the world, over 70 per cent of people with hypertension have poor or no control of their blood pressure, the situation is likely to be worse in other parts of the world including India. There are several reasons for this problem.

1. Even though the awareness and control of hypertension improved considerably between 1970 and 1990, studies have indicated that even in the US, increasing complacency is once again resulting in poor control of blood pressure.

2. Failure of doctors to understand and do their best in controlling hypertension.

3. Failure of the patients to understand the desirable level of blood pressure control. Controlling hypertension has long-term benefits. Patients are often interested only in short-term rewards and therefore fail to take treatment seriously.

4. High blood pressure does not usually cause symptoms, therefore many people fail to understand the real need for treatment.

5. Reluctance on the part of the doctor and the patient to prescribe or take more than one medication.

6. Failure to take medication altogether since most people with hypertension do not have any symptoms.

7. Problem of side effects of anti-hypertensive medications. A person with high blood pressure and no symptoms would naturally find it difficult to take medication if a particular drug caused side effects.

8. Failure to follow and comply with the lifestyle changes. Lifestyle changes (cessation of smoking, weight loss, exercise, dietary changes, etc.) are an important part of the treatment for a disease like hypertension. Although easy to understand, these changes are, in general, difficult to follow on a regular basis.

Whatever the reason, if you have high blood pressure and are either not taking any treatment or the blood pressure still remains high with your current medications, you need to do something about it as soon as possible. It is essential that both you and your doctor fully understand the risk of poor blood pressure control!

Remember, hypertension is a silent killer that will slowly and gradually damage your heart, kidneys and brain. Your arteries are being constantly damaged because of the excessive pressure exerted by high blood pressure. Why not get your blood pressure under control?

> 'If every physician could reduce systolic blood pressure by 2 mmHg in his patients, there would be a 6 per cent reduction in stroke mortality per year.'
>
> — *Ray W. Gifford, Vice-Chairman of Medicine, Cleveland Clinic, USA*

Consequences of High Blood Pressure

Apart from the high financial costs, the loss of life from the complications of hypertension is simply too difficult to calculate.

With rapid industrialisation, many of the advancing countries like India are facing a rising numbers of heart disease and stroke. High blood pressure remains the leading risk factor for both these conditions.

Premature Ageing and Damage to Arteries. You might wonder why it is important to control blood pressure if there are no symptoms or complaints. Remember, failure to control hypertension can only result in a less than optimal benefit for your health. As a result of high blood pressure, the heart has to work harder to pump the blood to other organs in the body. With each beat, if the heart is made to work harder because of the hypertension, the pressure and the changes in the blood vessels lead to premature hardening and narrowing of the arteries.

This in turn often results in damage to the brain (stroke), heart (heart attack), kidneys (kidney failure) or even the eyes (poor vision).

For example, it is estimated that a 15/10 mmHg rise in blood pressure above the desirable level of 140/90 mmHg doubles the risk of cardiovascular or kidney damage due to hypertension. In other words, if blood pressure remains close to 155/100 mmHg, the person is at twice the risk of these life-threatening complications.

Premature Death. Two of the leading causes of death in people over the age of 60 years are a heart attack and stroke, and both result from years of damage done to the arteries of the heart or the brain by high blood pressure. In almost all cases, experienced doctors would tell you that such complications are almost completely avoidable. If high blood pressure is controlled with appropriate treatment, such potentially fatal complications can be avoided. With better control of hypertension, the complications of hypertension have been reduced almost by half in the last 30 years in the United States. Even with this degree of success, much more requires to be done.

Undetected Disease. Many otherwise healthy looking people have hypertension. It is estimated that millions of adults remain undiagnosed for several years. The answer is very simple. If you do not already know your blood pressure readings, have your blood pressure checked within the next few days.

Benefits of Controlling Hypertension

As a direct result of better understanding and control of hypertension there has been a significant decline in the death rate due to stroke in the US and some other countries. Better blood pressure control is also believed to have contributed to a lower death rate due to coronary heart disease.

The benefits of treating hypertension have been repeatedly shown by various researchers from different countries including Australia, England, Sweden and the United States. Aggressive treatment of hypertension is essential for all adults, irrespective of their country or place of residence. Both the patient as well as the doctor must remain committed to a strict control of hypertension. In the United States, recently,

Northwestern Mutual Life Insurance estimated that an average person with untreated high blood pressure is likely to have his life span reduced by approximately 6 years. Adults with stage 1 hypertension and with very little symptoms are also likely to die prematurely if their blood pressure was left untreated.

Numerous scientific studies have shown the clear benefits of treating high blood pressure. Some of these are:

Improved Quality of Life. In scientific studies, the quality of life has been noted to be better with better control of hypertension. Results of the recent clinical studies were published in 1998 (Hypertension Optimal Treatment Trial or HOT study[1]). Lowering of blood pressure was reported to improve the mood and overall quality of life in middle-aged as well as elderly patients.

Benefits of Early Treatment. Dr Anderson from Sahlgrenska University Hospital in Goteborg, Sweden conducted a study involving 7495 men aged 47 to 54. Ninety per cent of these men who were noted to be hypertensive were treated and followed annually for a period of 24 years. Cardiovascular complications and deaths were much lower in those patients who were started on treatment in the earliest stage.

Benefits of Controlling Systolic Blood Pressure. O'Donnell and his colleagues reported in 1997 that even mildly high systolic blood pressure (140 to 159 mmHg) significantly increases the risk of heart disease in the elderly and therefore blood pressure must be controlled even if you are over the age of 65.

Starr and his associates reported in 1996 the result of their study of 603 older men and women, all between the ages of 70 and 88. Over a period of 4 years, they found a better survival rate in those whose systolic blood pressure was lower than 150 mmHg. People with systolic blood pressure over 150 mmHg had a much higher death rate due to hypertension related complications.

Benefits of Controlling Diastolic Blood Pressure. MacMahon and his colleagues in their meta-analysis study reviewed the combined result of 9 different studies involving a total of 420,000 patients followed for a period of 6 to 25 years. It was noted that 4,260 patients had died of heart disease and 599 patients had died of stroke. They concluded that if the diastolic blood pressure was higher by 5 mmHg on average, the risk of heart attack and stroke went up by 21 per cent and 34 per cent respectively.

In the Framingham study, a direct relationship was noted between diastolic blood pressure (the lower number) and deaths due to heart attacks. The higher the blood pressure, the higher the incidence of deaths due to heart attacks. As early as in 1961, Framingham researchers reported that hypertension increased the risk of heart disease. The results from the Framingham heart study have also revealed that patients with hypertension were at least 3 times more likely to die from sudden coronary deaths as compared to people with normal blood pressure.

Reduced Risk of Cardiovascular Disease in Diabetics. Tight blood pressure control was found to be beneficial in reducing the risk of premature cardiovascular disease in diabetic patients in the United Kingdom Prospective

Diabetes groups (UKPDS), published in the British *Medical Journal* in 1998.

Reduced Risk of Kidney Damage. Better blood pressure control was shown to significantly reduce the progress of kidney damage in diabetic patients in a report published in 1998 in *Diabetes Residents Clinical Practice* by Bakris and colleagues.

The need to bring your blood pressure below 140/90 cannot be overemphasized. Just adopting a half-hearted approach is not going to be helpful. Maybe you have already tried to lose weight and make other lifestyle changes. Maybe because of repeated failures, you have just given up. If so, redouble your efforts. Fortunately, even moderate success in changing your lifestyle, along with medication can help to keep your blood pressure under control.

Know your Risk of Heart Disease

For every medical condition, including hypertension and heart disease, it is very important to understand thoroughly the risk factors commonly responsible for the disease. For hypertension and heart disease there are several risk factors that significantly increase the chances of developing these conditions. Although hypertension can cause several complications, including stroke, heart failure and kidney failure, it is heart disease that is considered to be the most dangerous of all conditions.

Only through a better understanding of the risk factors can steps be taken to really try and reduce the risk of heart attack. In recent years, based on the risk factors, several scoring systems have been developed to find out the overall risk of a person for developing heart disease.

There have been several other modifications of the risk factor calculation systems over the past decade. However, all scoring systems have taken the three major risk factors — high blood pressure, high blood cholesterol and the history of smoking — into consideration.

In the United States, based on the famous Framingham Study, a six-step scoring system has most recently been developed, for men as well as women to calculate the total score indicating the risk of heart disease. Besides increasing age, history of smoking, total cholesterol and HDL cholesterol level, high blood pressure has been considered an important risk factor in both men and women. In conclusion, high blood pressure is a major risk factor for the development of heart attacks and heart diseases. Therefore, it is important to understand the consequences of uncontrolled hypertension and the need for strict control of high blood pressure.

References

1. Hansson L Zanchetti A, Carruthers SG, et al, for the HOT Study Group. Effects of intensive blood pressure lowering and low dose aspirin in patients with hypertension. Principal results of the Hypertension Optimal Treatment (HOT) randomized trial. Lancet. 1998; 351: 1755-1762.

11

What is Good Blood Pressure Control?

The health of the people is really the foundation upon which all their happiness and all their power as a State depend.

Benjamin Disraeli
1877

In the United States, there has been a significant reduction in hypertension related complications over the past 30 years. This major reduction in complications has been seen in the form of lower rates of heart attacks, strokes, and kidney failure. However, lately, it has been noted that a lot more needs to be done as far as blood pressure control is concerned. Periodical National Health and Nutrition Examination Surveys (NHANES) are conducted in the United States to monitor the trends in the awareness, treatment and control of hypertension. As is clear from the surveys over three different periods, the results of 1991 to 1994 have not been very encouraging.

The results from the three different periods are given in the table as below.

Trends in Control of High Blood Pressure[1]

	1976-80	*1988-91*	*1991-94*
Awareness	51%	73%	68.4%
Treatment	31%	55%	53.6%
Control	10%	29%	27.4%

National Health and Nurtrition Examination Surveys.

If in an educated country like the United States, the results are far from satisfactory, what about a country like India and other countries with a high illiteracy rates?

Control of hypertension remains poor in many countries around the world. In a recent presentation, Dr Serup Erdine[1] from the University of Istanbul in Turkey discussed that, because of rising life expectancy and people living longer, cardiovascular problems were becoming far more common. Dr Erdine argued that in the 1980s, the life expectancy of people in the developing countries was close to 50 years. Now, about 70 per cent of them are expected to live for approximately 75 years. It was also pointed out that about 50 per cent of the approximately 525 million people world-wide hypertension, live in developing countries. Three hundred million of them simply do not know that they have hypertension.

The problem of poor control of hypertension has also been highlighted by many other researchers around the world.

A comparison of good control of hypertension was presented as below.

Good Control of Hypertension: Some Comparisons

USA	27%
UK	12%
Canada	13%
France	33%
Italy	9%
Korea	9%
India	9%
Turkey	6.2%
Zaire	2.5%

What is the Ideal Level of Blood Pressure?

For many years scientists and doctors have tried to define the values of blood pressure readings that could be considered to constitute good control of blood pressure. As you can very well appreciate, if you have high blood pressure and are trying to lower it, your first step would be to find out what your goal should be.

The ideal blood pressure number has been a matter of debate for over 30 years. Some 15 to 20 years ago, doctors commonly accepted blood pressure readings of 150/95 mmHg as normal and therefore, simply reassured their patients with those kinds of readings. Without complicating the matter at the current time, our best understanding is to accept the recommendations of the U.S. Joint National Committee on Detection Evaluation and Treatment of Hypertension. Their message is simple and clear:

- You must get your blood pressure below 140/90 mmHg under all circumstances. This is for all people with normal kidney function and not suffering from diabetes mellitus.

- The target rate is to bring and keep the blood pressure below 130/80 mmHg, if you happen to have diabetes mellitus or poor kidney function. The committee further warned that in this select group of people, unless the goal of blood pressure control was achieved, the risk of complications remained much higher.

What does it all mean to you?

Remember that in the first instance, hypertension is a symptomless disease in most cases. Do not expect to experience any significant symptoms if blood pressure was 10 to 20 mmHg higher than the desirable 140/90 mmHg level. Yet, you should see your doctor soon. He or she may simply increase the dose of your current medications or change or add another type of tablet for better control of your blood pressure. Fortunately, with more than half a dozen different choices (diuretics, beta receptor blockers, ACE inhibitors, calcium channel blockers, alpha blockers, etc.) it cannot be that difficult to bring your blood pressure within the normal limits, i.e. below 140/90 mmHg.

You may have noticed that in most of my discussion so far, I have referred to the blood pressure readings of 140/90 mmHg as the cut-off point for good blood pressure control. However, there are several issues that are important to remember. Firstly, it is important to understand that this goal of 140/90 is only applicable to the general population with hypertension. For patients with kidney disease and diabetes mellitus, the goal is to keep the blood pressure below 130/85.

The US Joint National Committee on Detection, Evaluation and Treatment of Hypertension[2] has even revised its criteria for 'a good control' of hypertension in people with diabetes mellitus and/or kidney problems.

Good Blood Pressure Control in Renal Disease

Although the JNC VI advises that blood pressure be lowered to less than 130/85 mmHg in hypertensives with renal disease, some experts have argued for stricter control. In the Modification of Diet in Renal Disease Study[3], the researchers claim that only a tight blood pressure control of keeping the blood pressure below 125/75 mmHg can meaningfully delay progressive kidney damage in patients who already have a significant amount of protein loss in the urine (over 1000 mg of protein loss in 24 hours).

Good Blood Pressure Control in Diabetes Mellitus

In hypertensives with diabetes mellitus, researchers have similarly tried to study the role of intensive blood pressure control. In a report published in the *Archives of Internal Medicine* in September 2000, Dr Grossman and his colleagues concluded that strict blood pressure control was necessary to reduce the mortality and morbidity in hypertensives with coexisting diabetes mellitus. This study also reported that all four different types of commonly used medications (diuretics, beta blockers, calcium channel blockers and ACE inhibitors) were equally effective in controlling the blood pressure in diabetics and as long as the blood pressure remained satisfactorily under control, it did not matter what particular medication was being given to the patient.

Good Blood Pressure Control in Old Age

If you are over the age of 60 and have isolated systolic hypertension, then your systolic blood pressure should be kept below 140 and your diastolic between 70 and 90. Your doctor should, however, ensure that your diastolic blood pressure does not go below 65 since below this level your risk of complications could rise (see chapter 23).

Are Lower than Normal Readings Better for Health?

Based on the above facts you might argue that lower readings of blood pressure may even be better for good health. Why settle for 140/90 mmHg, 130/85 mmHg or even 120/80 mmHg as a marker for good control?

This question has been looked into by researchers especially in the Hypertension Optimal Treatment Study (HOT study)[4]. The HOT trial was uniquely designed to address the issue of how far blood pressure should be reduced to achieve the best benefits. This study included a total of 18,790 people with hypertension, between the ages of 50 and 80 from 26 different countries. Their diastolic blood pressures were tracked for a period of up to 3 years. It was mainly from this study that we learned that the maximum benefit was achievable when the diastolic blood pressure was brought down to close to 80 mmHg.

The message here is very simple: effective control of hypertension is essential to significantly reduce hypertension related complications, including heart disease and stroke.

Some experts in the past had argued that if the blood pressure was brought down too far, patients would be exposed to an increased risk of cardiovascular complications, including heart attacks. Many years ago, Cruickshank and his colleagues had first argued that if the diastolic blood pressure was brought down to 85-90 mmHg levels in hypertensives with already established coronary artery disease, these people were more likely to get heart attacks. This has been called as a J-curve phenomenon. These observations have, however, not been found to be true in other studies. In fact, the current consensus of expert opinion is that, if your blood pressure is not appropriately controlled, you remain at greater risk of suffering from heart disease, stroke and kidney failure.

While there has been some controversy regarding the ideal level of blood pressure, the following facts should help you to understand where your own blood pressure should be with proper treatment.

- In general your blood pressure should be kept below 140/90 mmHg.
- For those with diabetes mellitus or kidney disease, blood pressure needs to be kept below 130/80 mmHg.
- Those with evidence of protein urea with kidney disease (presence of protein in the urine) blood pressure should be kept below 125/75 mmHg.

References

1. Paper on 'Hypertension Control in Developing Countries' presented at the 18th Scientific Meeting of the International Society of Hypertension, Chicago, August 2000.
2. Chobanian AV, Bakris GL, Black HR, Cushman WC, Green LA, Izzo JL Jr, Jones DW, Materson BJ, Oparil S, Wright JT Jr, Roccella EJ; National Committee on Prevention, Detection, Evaluation and Treatment of High Blood Pressure, National Heart, Lung and Blood Institute; National High Blood Pressure Education Program Coordinating Committee, Seventh report of the Joint National Committee on Prevention, Detection, Evaluation and Treatment of High Blood Pressre, Boston University School of Medicine, Boston, Mass, USA. Hypertension. 2003 Dec' 42 (6): 1206-52.
3. Klahr S, Levey AS, Beck GJ, et al. The effects of dietary protein restriction and blood pressure control on the progression of chronic renal disease: modification of diet in renal disease study group. New England J Med 1994; 330(13): 877-884.
4. Hansson L, Zanchetti A, Carruthers SG, et al, for the HOT Study Group, Effects of intensive blood pressure lowering and low dose aspirin in patients with hypertension. Principal results of the Hypertension Optimal Treatment (HOT) randomized trial. *Lancet*, 1998; 351: 1755-1762.

12

Investigations for Hypertension

Mistakes live in the neighbourhood of truth and therefore delude us.

Rabindranath Tagore

High blood pressure being an asymptomatic disease, that is, it produces or shows no symptoms, in most cases, the diagnosis is made during a routine check-up at a doctor's clinic. It is important that before a final diagnosis is made, blood pressure be checked at least on three separate occasions with a reasonable interval of rest before each blood pressure reading.

All newly diagnosed patients with hypertension require certain baseline investigations. Although specialised and more sophisticated investigations may be necessary to confirm the secondary causes of hypertension, commonly performed tests for all hypertension patients are summarised in the table.

Laboratory Investigations

Tests	*Purpose*
Urine Analysis	To assess kidney function.
Sodium, Potassium, Calcium Levels	To confirm aldosteronism and Cushing's syndrome.
Blood Urea & Creatinine	To assess kidney function.
Blood Lipids	To rule out lipid abnormalities (HDL, LDL & triglyceride levels)
Blood Glucose	To rule out diabetes mellitus. Also helps to identify several secondary causes of hypertension.
Haemoglobin & Haematocrit	To check for a condition called polycythaemia causing hypertension, low haemoglobin may be seen in advanced renal disease.

High blood pressure, if left untreated, causes a lot of strain on heart. With progressive dilatation, the left ventricle (the main chamber that pushes the pure blood to the aorta and all parts of the body) becomes dilated and thickenend. ECG, chest x-ray and echocardiography can all help in determining the size of the left ventricle, i.e. the left ventricular hypertrophy.

ECG. An initial electrocardiogram is recommended for all patients with hypertrophy even if clinical examination may not indicate the presence of left ventricular hypertrophy. A baseline ECG recording is always very helpful for future monitoring of the effect of blood pressure on your heart. ECG is also needed to assess the heart rhythm, ischemic changes and hypertrophy.

Chest X-Ray. Chest X-ray can be helpful not only for detecting and confirming heart size enlargement, but also to rule out findings commonly associated with the coarctation of aorta, a condition responsible for a secondary type of hypertension. In coarctation of the aorta, the chest X-ray will show dilatation of the aorta with signs of rib notching. These findings, are of course, best left for the X-ray specialist (radiologist) and the doctor to diagnose.

Echocardiography. Although echocardiography is not considered necessary for all hypertension patients, it is a much better test than ECG for early detection of left ventricular hypertrophy. Many hypertension experts consider echocardiography as an appropriate and a cost effective investigation for hypertension.

Remember that in approximately 95 per cent of cases, the hypertension happens to be of the primary type with no single underlying cause. Secondary hypertension with a defined cause is seen in less than 5 per cent of cases. Many of the specialised investigations required for the detection of secondary causes of hypertension are available only in the major hospitals. If you are suspected of suffering from one of the secondary types of hypertension, the doctor may choose to refer you to a hypertension expert in a specialised medical centre/ hospital.

The doctor, to ascertain secondary hypertension may go in for specialised tests.

13

Consequences of High Blood Pressure

It is a poor government that does not realize that prolonged life, health and happiness of its people are its greatest asset.

Charles Horace Mayo
1919

You might ask that if high blood pressure in most cases does not produce symptoms, why should one bother at all to take any treatment? If it does not cause any pain, weakness or disability should an individual really be worried about the high blood pressure reading itself? The answer is a definite yes!

Over the years, if untreated, uncontrolled hypertension is not only a major risk factor for the heart but for other organs as well, including the vascular system, the brain, kidney, eyes, etc.

Coronary Heart Disease

It has been established beyond any doubt that both

systolic and diastolic hypertension raise the risk of heart attacks. It has also been noted that patients with hypertension have a far more serious outcome of heart attacks as compared to people with no history of hypertension.

Several complex mechanisms operate to produce the narrowing of the coronary arteries and the thickening of the artery walls in patients. These structural changes are more marked in hypertensives who also have other associated risk factors including smoking, high cholesterol, diabetes mellitus, obesity and lack of physical exercise.

The goal of hypertension control is to lower the risk of heart attack and reduce the progression of coronary heart disease. Some scientific studies have suggested that although the incidence of stroke is significantly reduced with a good control of blood pressure, the reduction in the rate of heart attack is somewhat smaller.

After a thorough evaluation, the doctor may choose to prescribe two or more agents to control your blood pressure. Beta blockers, ACE inhibitors and calcium channel blockers are some of the preferred choices in the case of an individual who has both hypertension as well as coronary heart disease (see chapter 17).

Heart Disease

The term heart disease is often used to describe any of the several diseases relating to the healthy working of the heart. These are briefly discussed here.

Left Ventricular Hypertrophy (LVH). Uncontrolled hypertension puts tremendous pressure especially on the left ventricle of the heart. The left ventricle is the major chamber of the heart which is responsible for pumping pure blood to the aorta, the main pipe through which the blood flows to all parts of the body via numerous arteries. In order to maintain sufficient blood supply in a person suffering from hypertension the left ventricle not only has to work harder but also against extra pressure and resistance. Several studies have confirmed that with poor blood pressure control, the left ventricle mass becomes much bigger, i.e., there is development of left ventricular hypertrophy. The extra stress and strain that the heart undergoes, because of the failure to control blood pressure is likely to lead to left ventricular hypertrophy, heart failure, heart attack and even sudden death.

LVH itself is associated with a higher risk of premature death. A patient with LVH is at a far greater risk of developing sudden abnormal and irregular heart beat (cardiac arrhythmia) and sudden death.

Normally, the better the blood pressure control the lower the chances of developing LVH. However, the

Hypertension and LVH: Facts to Remember

- LVH is a major problem associated with hypertension.
- For proper diagnosis of LVH you need to have an echocardiography.
- LVH raises the risk of congestive heart failure (CHF) and of premature death.
- LVH can be successfully reversed with medications and strict blood pressure control.
- Your doctor is the best person to advise you regarding the management of your blood pressure in the presence of LVH.

impact of high blood pressure is not always uniform in all patients. There is a degree of variability between patients but that does not mean that high blood pressure readings can be ignored. The law of physics almost always wins in all cases.

Tests for LVH. Since the presence of left ventricular hypertrophy is considered to increase the risk of death by 2 to 5 times, investigation is required to establish LVH. Chest X-ray, electrocardiography and echocardiography are three different tests that can help to determine the size of the left ventricle and establish the presence or absence of LVH. Echocardiography is considered to be the most sensitive test and is much better than electrocardiography in determining the size of the left ventricle. Echocardiography is widely available in most good hospitals. Many cardiologists even have an echocardiography machine available in their offices/clinics.

For a person suffering from hypertension it may be wise to have an echocardiography done in the near future. The findings of LVH itself should make you and your doctor think of re-evaluating your current plan of treatment.

Since the renin-angiotensin system and an overactive sympathetic nervous system are considered to play a significant role in causing LVH, your doctor may consider switching to ACE inhibitors or beta blockers — the two classes of medications that are most helpful in reducing LVH. Calcium channel blockers and diuretics are also considered to be a good choice for LVH. Some of the other medications such as vasodilators are not considered to be the favourable choices for the purpose of reducing the LVH.

Sudden Death. A variety of heart diseases may cause sudden death. In most cases the cause of sudden death is noted to be coronary heart disease. However, hypertension may also result in sudden death. Sudden death in hypertensive patients is associated with significant left ventricular hypertrophy which commonly results from uncontrolled hypertension. Along with left ventricular hypertrophy, hypertension also accelerates the risk of coronary artery disease. A combination of coronary artery disease and left ventricular hypertrophy (LVH) is usually responsible for sudden cardiac irregularity (arrhythmia) and sudden death.

Because of the possibility of sudden cardiac arrhythmias in patients with LVH, many experienced physicians strongly favour the use of beta blockers for the treatment of hypertension.

Angina Pectoris and Heart Attack. Coronary heart disease may be manifested as angina pectoris or an acute heart attack.

Over a period of time high blood pressure leads to the hardening and narrowing of all arteries including the arteries of the heart itself. This compromises the supply of blood to the heart muscles and the heart is deprived of sufficient blood and oxygen, especially when it has to beat a little faster. If you climb even one flight of stairs or run a short distance (10 to 20 metres) to catch the bus, your heart needs to beat faster in order to maintain enough blood supply to the muscles.

A person is said to have angina if during exercise he experiences chest pain. Typically, this type of chest pain disappears once you slow down and take rest. In other words, while at rest and not exercising, the coronary arteries are able to supply enough blood to the heart, but on exercising, when the heart beats faster to ensure sufficient blood supply, pain is experienced.

Some patients with advanced degree of coronary heart disease may experience the chest pain even at rest — unstable angina.

Congestive Heart Failure and Cardiomyopathy. Congestive heart failure or CHF is one of the major heart problems.

Shortness of breath on exertion, swelling of the legs and feet and tiredness are classical features of CHF. If you have one or more of these symptoms you should see your doctor as soon as possible.

As a result of long standing hypertension, the heart muscle is adversely affected. In almost all patients developing CHF due to hypertension, increased resistance to the emptying of the left ventricle leads to ventricular hypertrophy and subsequent dilatation (cardiomyopathy). Dr Marcos A. Rossi[1] demonstrated that years of chronic hypertension leads to the accumulation of collagen fibres in the heart muscle. It is this excessive collection of collagen tissue that eventually leads to the eventual stiffening and failure of the heart. CHF is often seen in hypertensive patients as they grow older. In some hypertensive patients with kidney failure, increasing fluid retention may put excessive load on the heart and cause CHF.

Ageing itself is associated with the weakening and loss of the cells of the heart (myocytes). Progressive cardiac dilatation and dystrophy of the heart simply leads to CHF.

Dr Daniel Levy, the Director of Framingham Heart Study recently reported that CHF has become a leading cause of hospital admission in the United States mainly because of an ageing population and hypertension. Unfortunately, despite a much better understanding of the development and treatment of CHF once it develops, the majority of patients are dead within 2 to 4 years.

CHF in the presence of hypertension requires aggressive treatment both for hypertension control as well as for management of CHF. In the past, digoxin and diuretics used to be the standard treatment for CHF. However, nowadays, ACE inhibitors and beta blockers are also considered to be an essential part of the comprehensive treatment of CHF. Fortunately, both beta blockers and ACE inhibitors are also commonly used for the control of hypertension.

In summary, uncontrolled hypertension may result in several serious and even life threatening cardiac complications. The single best approach is to prevent these complications by proper understanding and control of hypertension.

Complications of the Vascular System

High blood pressure has the potential to upset and disturb the normal and smooth working of the blood vessels which circulate the blood around the body. High blood pressure can cause the following complications:

Peripheral Vascular and Carotid Artery Disease. The normal blood vessels of a young person have a high degree of ability to relax and dilate. However, in hypertensive patients, these arteries gradually lose their ability to relax.

Medical research has established that this difficulty in dilating and relaxing the blood vessels is considered to play a major role in the vascular dysfunction and damage associated with hypertension.

In recent years, nitric oxide has been recognised to play a major role in the proper functioning of all blood vessels in the body. Further research in this field will almost certainly lead to a better understanding of hypertension and hypertension related vascular complications.

Atherosclerosis. Hypertension adversely affects the walls of the arteries as well as the smaller arterioles. Although the precise mechanism of this damage remains unclear, it is sufficient to understand that high blood pressure causes constant trauma and damage to the millions of blood vessels in the body. The walls of the vessels have millions of smooth cells that are constantly being damaged if the blood pressure remains high. Damaged cells become thick and excessive fibrous tissue is deposited on the walls of these vessels. Over a period of several years, calcium, cholesterol and fat deposition leads to progressive stiffening, narrowing and hardening of the arteries.

Progressive thickening and hardening of the arteries and arterioles is the basis for insufficient blood supply and damage to vital organs like the heart, brain and the kidneys.

Many of the changes that are usually considered to be a part of normal ageing occur at a much earlier age with hypertension. The state of your blood vessels, therefore, is the key to your health.

Peripheral Vascular Disease (PVD). The process of atherosclerosis affects almost all arteries in the body. One of the common medical problems is peripheral vascular disease. PVD patients have problems with the blood supply to the muscles of their legs and feet and often suffer from intermittent claudication which simply means that you have pain while walking, but the pain is relieved at rest. The hardening and narrowing of the arteries of the legs obstruct the blood flow in the leg muscles and therefore every time you walk, you end up with pain.

Carotid Arteriosclerosis. The carotid artery is a main blood vessel that runs on each side of the neck and supplies blood to the parts of the brain. If you have carotid arteriosclerosis, you may suffer from transient attacks of weakness of one or the other side of your body, with dizziness and even visual problems. The diagnosis, however, requires a thorough physical examination by the doctor. Not only does the blood pressure need to be properly controlled, but there may be need for further surgical procedures to relieve the obstruction to the blood flow in cases of significant carotid artery stenosis.

Carotid arteriosclerosis is commonly seen in people in their 60s and 70s especially if they have high blood pressure.

Aortic Aneurysm and Aortic Dissection. The walls of the aorta and other arteries have three distinct layers. The innermost layer is the intima, the middle layer is called the media and the outermost layer is called the adventitia.

As a result of constant trauma due to high blood pressure, a tear may develop in the intima. The tear may lead to the blood flowing through the layers of aorta, i.e. the dissection of the aorta. The aorta is a long tube that arises from the root of the heart and travels through the chest and enters the abdomen through the diaphragm, the big muscle that separates the chest from the abdomen. Depending upon the site of the damage, the dissection of the aorta may happen in the thoracic or the abdominal part of the aorta. Patients with aortic dissection require urgent medical attention. Unfortunately, over 50 per cent of patients die once they develop a dissection.

In most cases, patients with aortic dissection have a history of high blood pressure. Appropriate control of hypertension is, therefore, necessary to prevent the development of this life threatening complication.

The Effects of Hypertension on the Brain

Uncontrolled hypertension can have a debilitating effect on the brain. In the US deaths caused by the effects of uncontrolled high blood pressure on the brain ranks only behind deaths resulting from heart disease and cancer.

Stroke and Cerebrovascular Disease. Stroke is the third leading cause of death, heart disease and cancer being the first two, in the United States. Each year over 500,000 people are affected by stroke. In many other countries too, stroke is one of the five leading causes of disability and death.

It is also recognised that 90 per cent of all stroke victims have high blood pressure. In recent years, there has been a dramatic reduction in the rate of stroke in many countries as a result of better control of blood pressure. However, a lot more needs to be done, especially in developing countries where millions of patients with high blood pressure either remain undiagnosed or are walking around with uncontrolled hypertension.

How does high blood pressure raise the risk of stroke? In most cases, a blood clot in the brain is responsible for causing a stroke. Patients with hypertension are also more likely to get a blood clot in the heart or the carotid arteries. A part of this clot may dislodge and go to the brain (thromboembolism) and cause stroke.

As a result of high blood pressure, a person is also at a greater risk of developing small areas of dilated blood vessels commonly called aneurysms, that may suddenly rupture and cause a brain haemorrhage.

The other effects of uncontrolled hypertension on the brain are the hardening and narrowing of the arteries of the brain.

Does mild hypertension also increase the risk of a stroke? The Framingham Heart Study tried to answer this question. Observation for a period of 40 years of thousands of patients with mild hypertension showed that 30 per cent of all strokes occur in patients with mild hypertension. Since many of these patients tend to be the elderly, who have had mild hypertension for many years it becomes a matter of great importance to treat all cases of mild hypertension specially the elderly.

Transient Ischemic Attacks (TIAs) or Mini Strokes. Hypertension can also cause a problem of mini strokes (transient ischemic attacks or TIAs). In transient ischemic attacks, the blood supply to the brain may be temporarily interrupted because of a small embolus or clot in the brain. Patients with mini strokes may have transient weakness, visual or speech disturbance lasting for a few minutes to a few hours.

By definition, in a transient ischemic attack the neurological deficit must not last for more than 24 hours.

Dementia. With high blood pressure you run a significant risk of getting multiple TIAs. Remember that with each stroke or even mini stroke, you may end up with the loss of a small part of your grey matter in the brain. A condition called vascular or multi-infarct dementia may be seen as a result of multiple areas of loss of brain tissue. The development of this type of dementia and loss of brain function is another example of a serious complication of untreated hypertension.

Although a thorough history and physical examination by the doctor is very helpful, a CT testing of the brain is essential to establish the final diagnosis of multi-infarct dementia.

Cognitive Decline or Decline in Mental Functions. There is overwhelming evidence that uncontrolled hypertension is a threat to memory and mental functions, and everything possible must be done to maintain blood pressure under control.

In a recent issue of *Journal of the American Heart Association*, Dr Gary A. Ford of England reported that even mild to moderate hypertension may reduce mental alertness and awareness in older people, and since ageing itself is associated with a decline in mental functions, it is important that all older people with hypertension receive proper treatment to control their blood pressure.

Are all antihypertensive medications equally effective in preventing hypertension-related decline in mental functions? There are not too many scientific studies to answer this question at this stage. In one published report in the *Journal of The American Geriatric Society*, in 2000, Dr Stephanie S. Richards and her colleagues from the University of Pittsburgh School of Medicine, reported that ACE inhibitors, beta blockers and calcium channel blockers were the best choices for the prevention of mental decline.

Kidney Damage

The problem of hypertension causing kidney damage must be taken very seriously. There is little doubt that if blood pressure remains uncontrolled there is a high risk of kidney failure. Even with good control of hypertension, a small number of patients (less than 15 per cent) may still develop mild impairment of kidney functions[2].

A vast majority of end-stage renal failure patients have kidney damage either due to diabetes mellitus or due to hypertension or both. In the United States alone, currently there are over 200,000 patients with end-stage renal disease requiring regular kidney dialysis.

Before the development of diuretics, in the 1950s, kidney failure was a leading cause of death among patients with hypertension Fortunately, because of the availability of kidney dialysis and transplantation, and better treatment of hypertension, kidney failure patients continue to live longer than ever before. However, renal insufficiency is still a major threat to all patients with hypertension.

In most cases, the kidney function is likely to deteriorate only if blood pressure remains poorly controlled for a period of several months to years. Hypertension experts strongly recommend that blood pressure be controlled and maintained below 120/80 mmHg if there is any evidence of renal insufficiency, otherwise renal insufficiency may progressively deteriorate and result in renal failure.

In most patients with hypertension, kidney damage is a very slow process and may take many years. However, in patients with malignant hypertension with severe elevation of blood pressure (systolic readings over 200 and diastolic readings over 120), the kidney damage may develop rapidly in a matter of months.

Can appropriate control of hypertension slow kidney damage? The answer is a definite yes. In an annual scientific meeting of The American Society of Hypertension, Dr Ojo[3], a researcher from the University of Michigan, presented his results from a 10 centre renal study group. This study, which lasted for a period of four years, proved that with tight control of hypertension the microalbuminuria (a sign of early kidney damage) improved in a majority of patients.

Eye Damage and Poor Vision

High blood pressure can slowly damage the retina, the inner layer of sensitive neurons that are responsible for vision. The examination of the eyes is considered to be an essential part of a comprehensive physical exam for all hypertensive patients. Blurring and the irregularity of the optic disk and other changes (haemorrhages and exudates) are often suggestive of serious eye complications of hypertension.

Apart from the problem of retinopathy resulting from hypertension, the incidence of age-related damage to the area of vision (macular degeneration) is also noted to be higher in patients with hypertension. In the Framingham Heart Study, it was noted that those with hypertension had a far higher chance of developing macular degeneration.

In most cases, the eye damage is seen only in those who have had uncontrolled hypertension for a prolonged period of several years. Once again, maintaining good control of blood pressure is the only way to prevent such complications.

Sexual Dysfunction

Sexual function may be adversely affected in those who have high blood pressure. Healthy sexual functioning has a lot to do with appropriate blood supply to the sexual organs. If, as a result of premature narrowing and hardening of the arteries, the penile blood supply becomes impaired, it results in sexual impotence. It has become increasingly clear that hypertension itself, and not the medicines, may be the root cause of impotence resulting from impaired penile blood supply.

Hypertension also adversely effects the sexual function of women. In a study conducted by Dr Duncan and his colleagues from Cooperstown, New York[4] it was noted that hypertensive women were at least twice as likely to experience sexual dysfunction.

Since a higher percentage of hypertensive patients also tend to be depressed, the sexual dysfunction may sometimes be purely a part of depression. Altogether, if an individual has high blood pressure and is experiencing any degree of sexual dysfunction, the matter must be discussed with the doctor. All current medications must be brought to the attention of the doctor for a full evaluation of the problem. Several commonly used antihypertensive medications including beta blockers and diuretics are known to cause sexual dysfunction. While research is inconclusive, generally ACE inhibitors are considered better than beta blocker, diuretics and aldomet and cause minimal problems.

References

1. Rossi, Marcos A; Ramos, Simone G; Prado, Cibele M. Chronic inhibition of nitric oxide synthase induces hypertension and cardiomyocyte mitochondrial and myocardial collagen remodelling in the absence of hypertrophy. Journal of Hypertension. 21(5): 993-1001, May 2003.
2. Study reported in *The New England Journal of Medicine* (1989).
3. Phillips RA, Faulkner M, Gassman J, Jaen L, Kuesk JW, Norris K, Ojo A. Recruitment of African Americans with chronic renal insufficiency into a multicenter clinical trial: the african american study of kidney disease and hypertension. J Clin Hypertens (Greenwich). 2004 Aug; 6 (8): 430-6.
4. Duncan LE et al. Does hypertension and its pharmacotherapy affect the quality of sexual function in women? American Journal of Hypertension. June 2000. 13 (6 pt 1): 640-647.

14

How to Prevent Hypertension

When meditating over a disease, I never think of finding a remedy for it, but, instead, a means of preventing it.

Louis Pasteur
1884

It is a widely known fact that prevention is better than cure. Although this is true for almost all conditions, prevention is perhaps more relevant to some of those diseases for which we have a better understanding of the risk factors. Take the example of heart disease. We know that smoking, high cholesterol and high blood pressure are three of the major risk factors for the development of coronary heart disease. Yet, there are millions who continue to smoke. Many more fail to take any interest in lowering their cholesterol or high blood pressure.

It is unfortunate that despite all available knowledge, many of us fail to act and almost 'choose' to suffer from heart disease developing as a result of inaction. Studies have shown that despite repeated messages regarding the health benefits of diet and exercise, major reduction of death from coronary heart disease during the past 25 years has come from the advances in the treatment and not because of preventive steps. One study reported that although between 1980 and 1990 there were 127,000 fewer deaths from heart disease in the United States only 25 per cent of this decline was noted to be due to primary prevention and lifestyle changes; the remaining 75 per cent was mainly because of advancement in medical treatment.

Unfortunately, the current health care system in most countries is focussed only on the detection and treatment of diseases. The critics of the current health care delivery system in the United States, for example, constantly blame the government for spending less than 5 per cent of the billions of dollars ear marked for health care for the prevention of diseases.

Primary Prevention. Primary prevention and secondary prevention are two terms that are commonly used in medical literature. The steps you take to prevent the first heart attack are considered to be a part of primary prevention.

Secondary Prevention. Steps taken to prevent the second heart attack are considered to be a part of secondary prevention. Some steps, like cessation of smoking, control of high blood pressure and high cholesterol, are necessary for both primary as well as for secondary prevention of heart disease.

For a person who has had a heart attack, and has high blood pressure, tight control of hypertension must become a top priority. The risk of a second heart attack is definitely higher if blood pressure control remains inadequate. If you are a survivor of the first heart attack then blood pressure control is considered to be an important part of secondary prevention of heart attacks.

Steps to Prevent Hypertension

Hypertension is a condition that is considered to be preventable. Making sensible lifestyle changes is essential for all individuals. You are never too young or too old to adapt to healthy living habits!

Dietary Changes. Dietary changes can certainly help in lowering and keeping blood pressure within the normal range. Several scientific studies have shown the benefits of vegetarian diets. A Dietary Approach to Stop Hypertension (DASH) trial clearly demonstrated the benefits of diets that are rich in fruits, vegetables and whole grains. In another trial called Treatment of Mild Hypertension Study (TOMHS)[1], lifestyle changes were noted to play a significant role in the reduction of blood pressure. Foods low in saturated fat and calories, and high in potassium, have been noted to prevent the development of hypertension in these studies.

Keep your Weight Under Control. It has been accepted that weight control is perhaps the single most important step that an individual can take to prevent the development of hypertension.

Remember, overweight people are 2 to 6 times more likely to develop hypertension. It is estimated that between 20 to 30 per cent of all hypertension patients develop high blood pressure simply because of being overweight. If you are already overweight you can expect to see lower blood pressure readings simply by losing a few kilos of extra weight. Most people tend to gain weight in their middle years, but that is not to say that nothing can be done about it. You can certainly stop gaining the weight but only if you are careful about it.

Weight gain is not only bad for blood pressure but increases the risk of developing several other conditions including diabetes mellitus, osteoarthritis, coronary heart disease, gallstones and even cancer (see chapter 15).

Reduce your Salt Intake. Salt intake should be reduced as much as possible by everyone seriously interested in lowering blood pressure. High salt and sodium consumption leads to the development of hypertension. Since many poor food habits start in childhood, parents can play an important role in keeping children from developing poor eating habits. Salt can be substantially reduced in cooking. The use of table salt must be kept to a minimum. Many types of snacks are usually loaded with extra salts and should be avoided (see chapter 15).

Reduce Stress. Excessive psychological stress is not good for health, including blood pressure. Do not always push yourself to the limit. Don't get into a situation where you are constantly on the run or trying to meet or beat deadlines. If you think you have type A personality, then try to change yourself into a type B personality. If stress is your major problem, try to read at least one or two good books on stress and stress management techniques (see chapter 15).

Engage in Regular Physical Exercise. Regular physical activity provides several benefits particularly for cardiovascular health. Adults with sedentary habits can expect to see a drop of 5 to 10 mmHg if they start to engage in regular aerobic type of physical exercise. Twenty to thirty minutes of moderate exercise at least five days a week is considered to be reasonable. Fortunately it does not have to be a strenuous form of exercise; moderate intensity is as good as strenuous exercise. If you believed in the no pain, no gain dictum, please change your mind (see chapter 15).

Increase your Potassium Intake. High potassium intake has been linked to lower blood pressure readings (see chapter 15).

Alcohol only in Moderation. While the consumption of 1 to 2 drinks per day of alcohol (beer, wine or whisky) has been shown to reduce the risk of cardiovascular disease, excessive alcohol intake is bad not only for blood pressure but for overall health. It is estimated that between 5 to 10 per cent of adults have hypertension because of excessive drinking. If you are a teetotaler, do not start drinking. If you are already used to your moderate drinking status (1 to 2 drinks per day), continue with your drinking but if your blood pressure has been high in the past or is currently high, limit your drinks to only one per day. Do not even go for a second drink. For some people even two drinks can become too much (see chapter 15).

References

1. Neaton JD, Grimm RH Jr, Prineas RJ, Stamler J, Grandits GA, Elmer PJ, Cutler JA, Flack JM, Schoenberger JA, McDonald R, et al. Treatment of Mild Hypertension Study. Final results. Treatment of Mild Hypertension Study Research Group. Division of Biostatistics, School of Public Health, University of Minnesota 55414. JAMA. 1993 Aug 11; 270 (6): 713-24.

15

Lifestyle Changes

The only way to keep your health is to eat what you don't want, drink what you don't like and do what you would rather not.

Mark Twain
1897

Healthy lifestyle habits — ideal body weight, regular exercise and proper diet — have been known for many centuries to be beneficial for good health. However, Western medicine has been slow to appreciate the role of these seemingly 'small' factors. The mind-body connection, for example, has only been accepted in Western medicine in the past 15 to 20 years.

What do we really mean by Lifestyle Changes?

When we talk about lifestyle changes do me mean not waking up early and continuing to sleep until late in the morning? Do you really have to take boiled vegetables, rice and lentil soup for the rest of your life if you happen to have high blood pressure? Does it mean that you must never have a cup of coffee or a glass of beer or wine? Does it mean that you must discard the use of salt altogether from your diet? Certainly not! Some of the sensible changes that are specifically considered to be helpful for the appropriate control of hypertension are giving up smoking, regular physical exercise, reduction of salt, following a low fat diet, weight reduction, reducing stress and keeping alcohol intake moderate.

Although many of these changes may appear to be 'no big deal', and just 'small sins', the total effect of poor lifestyle habits can add up and make the management of hypertension very difficult.

I have personally dealt with many patients whose idea of a healthy lifestyle is limited to low fat milk and just taking the stairs instead of using the elevator in a two-storey building. Many of these patients continue to smoke and indulge in high fat diets. No wonder at every followup clinic appointment, their blood pressure is noted to be high requiring increasing doses of medication. Yet, it is wrong to assume that lifestyle changes are easy to achieve. I have met many otherwise very intelligent and educated persons, including doctors, who, despite being very aware of the need for one or more lifestyle changes, have simply failed to do so.

Role of Lifestyle Changes

The role of lifestyle changes in the reduction of blood pressure has been reported by many researchers.

The Joint National Committee of US on Detection, Evaluation and Treatment of High Blood Pressure in its most recent report has strongly emphasised the role of lifestyle changes for the control of all grades of hypertension. Not only that, the committee also recommended some of the basic lifestyle modifications in order to prevent the development of hypertension.

In the United States, innovative programmes based on diet, exercise and stress reduction have been developed, and with these lifestyle changes, Dr Dean Ornish and his colleagues have been able to show that up to 77 per cent of patients with proven coronary heart disease could be saved from invasive heart procedures such as angioplasty or bypass heart surgery.

Even if there is no formal programme run by a nearby hospital do not be disheartened. With simple and sensible lifestyle changes discussed in this chapter you can expect to gain the same benefits. People are, of course, living longer in most parts of the world because of improvements in detection and treatment of diseases. There is no arguing that a healthy lifestyle can improve general health and lead to a better life expectancy.

A recent *Time* magazine article claimed that even if you have been ignoring your health for many years, you can still undo the damage and expect to avoid heart disease, diabetes mellitus and even cancer in your later years of life through lifestyle modifications.

Benefits of Lifestyle Changes

What type of benefits can you really expect with lifestyle changes as far as blood pressure control is concerned? There are several scientifically proven benefits for blood pressure that come with better lifestyle changes. You are less likely to develop hypertension. For someone who has hypertension, the control of blood pressure is likely to be better. With better control of your blood pressure, one may even be able to reduce the current doses of medications or even stop one or two types of tablets altogether. For someone who has mildly high blood pressure, there is a good chance of bringing it within the normal range even without the use of any kind of medicines.

There are numerous other added advantages of healthy lifestyle changes. Many of the other benefits are listed in the following table.

Benefits of Lifestyle Modifications

Problem	*Comments*
Obesity	Loss of body weight will help control blood pressure, cholesterol and reduce the risk of diabetes and heart disease.
High cholesterol	Regular exercise and dietary changes can reduce cholesterol.
Coronary heart disease	Healthy lifestyle changes can reduce the overall risk of heart disease.
Diabetes mellitus	A proper diet, regular exercise and weight control can cut down your risk of diabetes mellitus.
Osteoarthritis	Physical exercise and weight loss can help arthritis.
Bronchitis/ Emphysema	Lung functions improve with the cessation of smoking.
Stroke	Dietary changes, low fat intake, regular exercise and weight control reduce the risk of stroke.
Cancers	The risk of breast, prostate and other cancers is higher in people taking high fat diets and who are obese.
Depression/ Anxiety	Regular exercise improves the mood and lowers the risk of developing depression.

With numerous benefits of lifestyle changes, let us now look at these lifestyle modifications a little more in detail.

Essential Lifestyle Changes

Successful control of hypertension requires the combined efforts of the doctor and the patient. Medication do not and cannot suffice. A major and an active role has to be played by the patient by changing the lifestyle — losing weight, quitting smoking, if a smoker, observing strict control in alcohol consumption, reducing stress and adopting healthy eating habits.

Smoking. As a lifestyle change, the decision to stop smoking must receive top priority. Although, in the control of hypertension, cessation of smoking may not have a major role in reducing blood pressure, but it is important to remember that the goal in the control of hypertension is to prevent the ultimate problem of coronary heart disease. Unless smoking is stopped this goal is likely to remain elusive.

The British Medical Research Council Working Party in its report of 1985 concluded that patients with hypertension who continued to smoke are 3 to 5 times more likely to die of coronary heart disease as compared to non-smokers. Hypertension is often noted to be far more serious and of a malignant nature in those who smoke.

For someone who has high blood pressure and continues to smoke, the blood pressure control is likely to be poor despite taking medication. The level of hormones like adrenaline and nor adrenaline in the blood goes up with smoking. These chemical substances may also cause irregular heartbeats and sudden death, especially in patients whose heart muscles have already been adversely affected by years of hypertension.

If you have been smoking for many years, you can still stop and be rewarded with the many benefits. The good news is that the risk of sudden death is reduced substantially within a few weeks of giving up smoking. The flexibility and elasticity of the blood vessels improves once nicotine stops damaging the arteries.

Alcohol. Alcohol has a pressure effect in your body. There are many people who have mild to moderately high blood pressure simply because they drink too much. In some cases, if blood pressure is not controlled or is poorly controlled inspite of medications, alcohol may need to be completely stopped in order to bring blood pressure under control. Studies have indicated that blood pressure of an adult taking more than 3 to 4 drinks per day, is likely to be higher by 5 to 10 mmHg on average. Generally speaking, the greater the number of drinks, the higher will be the increase in blood pressure.

Medically speaking, a person with moderate drinking habits must not take more than 1 oz. of ethanol per day which approximately equals:

- 8 oz. of wine (250 ml approx.)
- 2 oz. of liquor (60 ml approx.)
- 24 oz. of beer (750 ml approx.)

How much is enough? What can you really expect by cutting down on drinks? Should you stay away from alcohol completely? Did you not hear recently that those who are light drinkers are less likely to die from heart disease? Yes, of course. Light drinking is considered to be helpful to your health. Here are some simple rules based on our current understanding of scientific research and studies.

1. In adults taking only one drink per day, the blood pressure was noted to be comparable to that of non drinkers.

2. If you are not a drinker, do not start drinking under the belief that it will save you from heart disease. The fact is that despite the recognised cardiovascular benefits of light drinking, too many people lose a balanced approach to alcohol and unfortunately end up with problems associated with alcohol abuse.

3. If you have already been drinking between 1 to 2 drinks per day and your blood pressure is well controlled with medications, you may continue to drink. However, be cautious and if possible, give up your second drink. Your chances of a better control of hypertension are much higher by exercising control.

Several studies have confirmed that light drinking is good for cardiovascular health and may, indeed, significantly cut down risk of heart disease. With scientific

Some ways to cut down your Drinking

- Try to take small sips.
- Take non alcoholic drinks.
- Try mixed drinks with a lower alcohol content.
- Don't give in to social pressure.
- Learn to say 'no' to the next drink.
- Avoid parties or places where you are likely to indulge in heavy drinking.

facts favouring the benefits of light drinking, it is hard to argue against the advantages of limited alcohol intake.

Too Much Stress is Dangerous. Psychological stress not only makes you feel tense, anxious and nervous but may also raise your blood pressure by activating the sympathetic nervous system. The well known fight or flight response consists of a situation where the person is dealing with a stressful situation and as a part of the psychological response the glands suddenly secrete an excessive amount of adrenaline. With excessive adrenaline secretion, the middle layer of artery walls, the medis, contracts excessively, causing the blood pressure to rise.

Unfortunately, some people tend to over-react and are noted to have an exaggerated cardiovascular response. Such individuals are classified as 'hot reactors'. Studies both in animals as well as in human beings have reported that the hot reactors — people with exaggerated response — are more likely to develop hypertension and coronary heart disease.

A stressful lifestyle and type A personality are commonly associated with numerous health hazards such as: increased risk of high blood pressure, difficulty in controlling hypertension despite taking treatment, increased risk of heart attack and increased risk of sudden death.

Stress and Modern Diseases. A straight forward simple fact: Psychological stress is perhaps your number one enemy. It has been argued that over 80 per cent of all modern day diseases are stress related. How can you, then, reduce your stress level? Is it possible to be completely free of stress? Perhaps, no. Yet, a lot can be

Type A and Type B Personalities

In 1959, Drs Freedman and Rosenman in California, were the first physicians to suggest that almost everyone could be divided into two distinct groups with different personalities called type A or type B personalities.

You can, in fact, ask yourself a few questions and be able to decide for yourself which category you fall into.

Type A Personality

- Wants to accomplish more and more in less and less time.
- Always in a rush.
- Feels that everybody is really too slow for him/her.
- Finds it difficult to wait in a line at the post office or anywhere else.
- Constantly trying to save time.
- Tries to do 2 to 3 activities at one time.
- Feels guilty for relaxing for a few hours.
- Feels that progress can be achieved through the fast lane alone.
- Weighs everything in terms of 'numbers'.

Type B Personality

- Believes in the virtue of patience.
- Can relax and do nothing for days without feeling guilty.
- Maintains a sense of calmness.
- Has no characteristics of type A personality.

done to lower stress levels. In recent years, yoga and meditation have been adopted as a way of life by millions across the world. Dean Ornish, an internationally recognised heart expert has demonstrated that heart disease can even be reversed with yoga, meditation and dietary changes. In his own book *Reversing the Heart Disease*, Dean Ornish admits that many of these lifestyle changes he incorporated in his own life after a visit to India. Biofeedback and regular exercise have been similarly shown to provide benefits in lowering the blood pressure.

For any stress management programme to work, it is important to identify the reason or reasons causing the stress. In most cases, people need to develop their own ways to relax. What may work for one person may not work for another. In any case, there is a lot of convincing evidence that regular relaxation techniques, lower blood pressure by an average of 5 to 15 mmHg.

Reducing Stress with Meditation. Although there is some continuing controversy regarding the precise role of and degree of response to meditation and other relaxation techniques in blood pressure treatment, most authorities recognise the positive role of stress and blood pressure reduction through these techniques.

Reduced Salt Intake: An Essential Change. Dr Norman Kalplan, a world-renowned heart specialist at the University of Texas, states that low salt intake is a simple lifestyle change that is really essential for treatment of all patients with hypertension.

Unfortunately we also know that physicians do not routinely discuss the question of salt sensitivity if blood pressure is within normal limits. Yet, as a general rule, it is in everyone's interest to lower the salt intake with age. Why? Because your blood pressure is likely to rise with normal ageing so why not do yourself a favour and start cutting down the salt intake from now onwards.

If you have high blood pressure, perhaps you have already been advised by your doctor to cut down on your salt intake. Is salt intake, then, the cause of hypertension? Unfortunately, it is not such a simple question to answer. Physicians and scientists have been studying the relationship between high blood pressure and salt intake for many years. It has been noted that societies with high salt consumption tend to have high blood pressure readings. In recent years, with increasing consumption of fast foods, the salt intake of most people with a fast pace of life has gone up. The American guidelines recommend that the daily salt intake should be kept under 6 grams per day but the average consumption in the US is 9 grams.

It is important to understand that even without added salt (table salt), most foods have salt (sodium) as their natural content. In fact, our body requires no more than 1.25 grams of salt per day for the proper functioning of the tissues. While processed foods are a source of 80 per cent of dietary salt in countries like the United States, in India excessive consumption of salt in the condiments (for example, pickles) is a major cause of high salt intake.

The Effects of High Salt Intake. High salt intake is believed not only to cause a rise in blood pressure but also to increase the risk of stroke. In the editorial published in *The Archives of Internal Medicine,* February 26, 2001 the world renowned cardiologist Frazn H. Messerli from

New Orleans, stated that there was a strong link between high salt intake and the high incidence of stroke, kidney damage and left ventricular hypertrophy, even if the blood pressure rise was minimal. In view of these dreadful consequences, the author of this editorial has recommended that all adults should try to reduce their salt intake as much as possible.

The effects of reducing salt intake has also been studied as a part of the famous DASH diet.

A group of 412 patients with an average age of 48 were studied. It was noted that when the patients from the high sodium (3300 mg) were switched to the low sodium group (1500 mg), their systolic and diastolic blood pressures went down by 6.7 and 3.5mm respectively. Once again, based on these scientific results, the authors of this widely recognised dietary approach study have strongly suggested that adults must not take more than 1500 mg of salt per day.

There is no simple test to find out whether you are a salt sensitive person or not. However, if your blood pressure has failed to come under control despite taking 2 to 3 different medications, you need to restrict your salt intake. The first step would be to stop taking any added table salt. Salted peanuts and potato chips may result in excessive intake of salt. If so, you know what to do. Fortunately, there are some salt substitutes that you can use instead of common salt. These substitutes contain potassium instead of sodium.

Salt Sensitivity. Because of the relationship of high salt intake and hypertension, salt sensitivity has become an increasingly interesting topic for researchers in recent years. Salt sensitive people do not always develop hypertension, i.e., there are many people with normal blood pressure readings and yet they are noted to be salt sensitive. In one study conducted by Dr Myron H. Weinberger over a period of 30 years it was noted that those who were salt sensitive had a very high risk of death due to cardiovascular problems. This was true despite the fact that their blood pressure levels remained within normal limits. Adults with high blood pressure and salt sensitivity were, of course, noted to be at a much greater risk of death as compared to salt sensitive adults with normal blood pressure readings. The conclusion was that salt sensitivity itself is a risky problem for your health.

Even though the role of lower salt intake remains somewhat inconclusive, most experienced physicians agree that lowering the salt intake can prove to be helpful in controlling blood pressure. It has been argued that approximately 50 per cent of all adults are salt sensitive and therefore they react very well to lower salt intake. In other words, lower salt intake helps them to reduce blood pressure.

Unfortunately, there is no simple test to determine whether you are salt sensitive or not. The only practical way to find out whether lower salt intake will help you lower your blood pressure is to go on a low salt diet for a period of 6 to 10 weeks and see the impact of this change on your blood pressure for yourself. You may be pleasurably surprised to see that your blood pressure is better controlled on the lower salt diet.

Reducing salt intake is likely to help in following ways:

1. If blood pressure is high-normal, cutting down on salt intake will help to keep blood pressure within the normal range. Since most people with high-normal blood pressure readings eventually develop hypertension, it is in their best interest to limit the salt intake and avoid the problem of hypertension.

2. If blood pressure is already high, reducing salt intake will help to lower the blood pressure by 5 to 10 mmHg. In some cases of mildly elevated blood pressure, it may even be possible to keep it within the normal range and discontinue or reduce antihypertensive medication being taken. The decision to change or discontinue the medication must be made by the doctor.

3. If blood pressure has not been adequately controlled even with medication, simply cutting down on salt can help to achieve blood pressure control.

Use the following Herbs and Spices instead of Salt

with tomatoes	: Garlic, onion, parsley, basil
with carrots	: Parsley, green pepper, onion, tomato, chilly powder
with green beans	: Thyme, nutmeg, onion, lemon
with potatoes	: Parsley, onion, mace (*javitri*)
with fish	: Lemon, garlic, basil (*tulsi*)
with meat	: Bay leaves (*tejpatta*), thyme leaves (a variety of *pudina*), onion, dry mustard, parsley (*ajmood*)
with pork	: Fresh/dried celery leaves, parsley, thyme

All of us, irrespective of our blood pressure levels, must use salt sparingly and choose our foods carefully. To help you in this selection we give below the foods which you should have and those which should be avoided.

Persons on Low Salt Diet must avoid

Table Salt

Meats

- Salted/smoked meats
- Bacon
- Ham
- Sausages
- Luncheon meats and frankfurters

Fish

- Salted/preserved fish
- Sardines

Snack Foods

- Potato chips
- Pretzels
- Salted peanuts, almonds, cashew
- Salted popcorn
- Fried *namkeen (samosa, kachori)*

Condiments

- Pickles/*chutneys*
- Olives
- Ketchup
- Soy sauce
- Chilli sauce, other similar sauces and mustard etc.

Dairy Foods

- All cheeses
- Whole milk
- Ice cream
- Salted *laasi*

Vegetables

- Tomato juice (canned)
- Lima beans (frozen)
- Peas (frozen)
- Spinach (canned)
- Carrots (canned)
- Salads with excessive salt

Miscellaneous

- Baking soda
- Baking powder
- *Chappaties* with added salt

Persons on Low Salt Diet can have

Fruit

Apples
Apricots
Bananas
Cantaloupe
Dates
Grapefruit
Melons
Prunes
Raisins
Watermelon

Fruit Juices

Apple juice
Grapefruit juice
Prune juice
Orange juice

Fresh Vegetables

Asparagus
Barley
Carrots
Cabbage (cooked)
Corn
Cucumber
Cauliflower (cooked)
Green beans (cooked)
Green pepper
Lettuce
Mushrooms
Beans
Onions
Peas (cooked)
Potatoes (baked/ boiled)
Spinach
Tomatoes
Turnip (green)
Frozen vegetables without salt and
Corn on the cop

Meats

Chicken/Other poultry
Liver

Fresh Fish

Cereal Products

Bread or chappaties made without salt or with sodium-free baking powder
Shredded wheat
Rice

Dairy Products

Non-fat dry milk
Skim milk
Unsalted margarine

Beverages

Coffee and Tea
Lemonade

Spices

Garlic
Pepper
Onion powder
All spices that do not contain salt

Physical Exercise

It is a recognised fact that regular physical exercise helps to lower blood pressure. People with a sedentary lifestyle are at a much greater risk of developing hypertension than those who exercise regularly. The combined effects of exercise and weight loss can make a significant difference in keeping blood pressure under control. The US Joint National Committee report on hypertension has emphasised the need for regular physical activity for all patients with hypertension. Fortunately, there is no need to indulge in strenuous exercise in order to gain the cardiovascular benefits of lowered blood pressure and reduced risk of heart disease. Regular aerobic exercise has been noted to reduce blood pressure between 5 and 10 mmHg.

In cases where blood pressure is totally uncontrolled at the present time medical advise must be sought without delay. One must not become a victim of laziness or procrastination.

When to Exercise. Questions have often been raised regarding the best time of day for physical exercise. These days it is common to find people engaging in physical exercise at almost any time of the day. Most health clubs are open from early morning to late at night.

Generally speaking, it is best to avoid physical exercise 1 to 2 hours after main meal or before bedtime. Since exercise increases circulation and mental alertness, there may be some difficulty in sleeping if you have been exercising 1 to 2 hours before sleeping. Since systolic blood pressure is normally higher in the early morning hours, some people are afraid of pushing their blood

Some helpful Exercises

Type of Exercise	*Calories Burnt per hour*
Running	650
Basketball	650
Football	540
Rope skipping	580
Swimming	490
Cycling	380
Walking	230
Fishing	250
Bowling	300
Table Tennis	280

pressure still higher with exercise in the morning hours. However, studies have reported that physical exercise in hypertensive patients in the early morning hours is as safe as at any other time of the day.

The Benefits of Exercise. Physical exercise is beneficial for hypertension in several different ways, including reducing the stiffness of the arteriolar walls, improving insulin sensitivity and decreasing stress hormones. The continued effect of these rather complex changes results in lowering the blood pressure.

What about isometric or muscle strengthening exercises for patients with hypertension? Although intense isometrics exercise such as weight-lifting commonly cause the blood pressure to rise, repetitive weight training with moderate weights has no adverse effects.

Regular exercise has numerous other advantages for general health and well being. It leads to lowering of blood pressure, weight reduction, decreases the risk of heart attack, and diabetes mellitus. Exercise also, reduces bad (LDL) cholesterol and increases your good (HDL) cholesterol. It helps to control blood sugar even in diabetics, makes bones stronger and prevents osteoporosis. Physical exercise is known to improve the mood, sleep and general energy level, and reduce anxiety, depression and stress. It keeps you young and cheerful.

Different types of exercises are associated with different calorie-burning power.

Can Physical Exercise be Dangerous or even cause Sudden Death? Occasionally you will hear about someone who went jogging or was involved in some strenuous exercise and died suddenly while exercising. Is there a real reason to be scared of joining an exercise programme? The answer is a definite no!

The risk of sudden death while exercising is almost negligible for most people. Most sudden deaths happen in those who have had a sedentary lifestyle and suddenly one day decide to go for a strenuous exercise. That can certainly put too much burden on the heart. In some cases, sudden death has been noted in persons who previously had an unrecognised heart problem. Therefore, if you have not been previously exercising and plan to

> The following steps can prove helpful in controlling your body weight.
>
> - Cut down your total caloric intake.
> - Cut down your fat intake.
> - Go for regular exercise.
> - Replace high calorie snacks with low calorie food.
> - Maintain a food diary that can help monitor your eating behaviour.

exercise in the near future, a thorough physical examination (including your blood pressure measurement and examination of the heart) by your doctor is strongly advised. This is more important if you are over the age of 40 and happen to have a family history of high blood pressure or heart disease. In some cases the doctor may even decide to perform an exercise stress test before giving a clean bill of health.

If your blood pressure is satisfactorily controlled, you can engage in most types of physical exercise. A sensible plan of aerobic exercise (30 to 40 minutes per day for most days of the week) would be more helpful in lowering blood pressure. However, it is best to check with your doctor before any serious physical exercise programme is started.

16

Diet and Weight Control

We eat too much, drink too much, smoke too much, drive too fast, and walk too little.

Margaret C. Heagarty
1976

Obesity has long been known to be related to a rise in blood pressure. Weight reduction has been commonly recommended to prevent the development of hypertension in people with high-normal blood pressure. Similarly, in obese hypertensive patients, weight reduction is considered to be a desirable goal. Both systolic and diastolic blood pressures rise with increasing body weight.

In the Framingham Study, the risk of hypertension was noted to be 3 to 10 times higher in people from the most obese group as compared to those with normal body weight. The Bogalusa Heart Study researchers also confirmed that obese children had a much higher incidence of hypertension.

In a recent study, Alison Field and her colleagues from Harvard Medical School reported (*Archives of Internal Medicine, July 9, 2001*) the relationship between being overweight and obese with several common chronic diseases. During their ten-year follow-up of adults, they noted that the incidence of diseases including diabetes mellitus, hypertension, heart disease, stroke, colon cancer and gallstones rose significantly as they continued to gain excessive body weight.

Since weight loss has been shown to reduce blood pressure, control of obesity is considered to be one of the major lifestyle modifications necessary. In recent years, it is becoming clear that central obesity (too much fat deposited around the tummy area) is perhaps the root cause of several health problems. It has been postulated that with central obesity, people develop insulin resistance, high blood pressure, high cholesterol, diabetes and heart disease.

Ideal Height/Weight. Before we discuss the problem of obesity and excessive weight further, it is important to give you some idea about your own body weight. The body weight chart as developed by the Life Insurance Corporation of India provides the desirable body weight for Indian men and women given on the next page.

Ideal Height/Weight Chart Without Shoes

Height			Weight	
Men 25+ years				
Ft	*In*	*Cm*	*lbs*	*Kg*
5	2	157.5	118-129	53.5-58.5
5	3	160.0	121-133	54.9-60.3
5	4	152.6	124-136	56.2-61.7
5	5	165.1	127-139	57.6-63.0
5	6	167.6	130-143	59.0-64.9
5	7	170.2	134-147	60.8-66.7
5	8	172.7	138-152	62.6-68.9
5	9	175.3	142-156	64.4-70.8
5	10	177.8	146-160	66.2-72.6
5	11	180.3	150-165	68.0-74.8
6	0	182.9	154-170	69.9-77.1
6	1	185.4	158-175	71.7-79.4
6	2	188.0	162-180	73.5-86.6
Women 25+ years				
4	10	147.3	96-107	43.5-48.5
4	11	149.9	98-110	44.5-49.9
5	0	152.4	101-113	45.8-51.3
5	1	154.9	104-116	47.2-52.6
5	2	157.5	107-119	48.5-54.0
5	3	160.0	110-122	49.9-55.3
5	4	162.6	113-126	51.3-57.2
5	5	165.1	116-130	52.6-59.0
5	6	167.6	120-135	54.4-61.2
5	7	170.2	124-139	56.2-63.0
5	8	172.7	128-143	58.1-64.9
5	9	175.3	132-147	59.9-66.7
5	10	177.8	136-151	61.7-68.5
5	11	180.3	140-155	63.5-70.3
6	0	182.9	144-159	65.3-72.0

Source: Life Insurance Corporation of India

Body Mass Index. Although the weight chart is generally very helpful, a better way to find out whether you are obese or not is to determine your Body Mass Index (BMI). BMI takes into account both your height and weight in determining whether there is excess fat. The formula to calculate BMI is:

How to Calculate your Body Mass Index (BMI)

$$\text{Body Mass Index} = \frac{\text{Weight in kg}}{(\text{Height in metres})^2}$$

	Ideal	*Overweight*	*Obese*
BMI for Men	17-25	25-30	>30
BMI for Women	17-27	27-32	>32

Achieving Weight Control

Weight control is usually achieved through two principle mechanisms.

1. A change of dietary habits to achieve a lower intake of calories.

2. Starting a regular exercise regimen to achieve a higher calorie utilisation or expenditure.(See chapter 15).

In simple terms, weight control is very much like a personal bank account. You will surely have more money in it if you keep depositing and spending only very little. This simple concept applies to body weight as well. If a person keeps on eating (intake of calories) and has a sedentary lifestyle (too little expenditure of calories) with practically no exercise, the chances of becoming overweight are very high.

Obesity is almost an epidemic in many countries around the world, including some developing countries, where obesity is being increasingly noticed in the affluent urban population. No wonder almost every household in big Indian cities has at least 1 to 2 adults with common lifestyle diseases such as hypertension, diabetes mellitus and heart disease. Obesity is certainly a chronic disease that is multifactorial in origin. Genetic factors leading to hereditary inheritance of obesity is commonly accepted as a major problem since obesity seems to run in families. Anxiety and/or depression may also lead to overeating and weight gain.

Weight Loss through Behaviour Modification. In Western societies millions of dollars are spent on dieting and weight loss programmes. Is dieting only a matter of will power? This has been a matter of continuing debate for many years. Many Western scientists currently hold the view that will power alone has very little to do with dieting and it is only through behaviour modification that people can achieve a meaningful weight loss. If you wish to really lose weight through dieting, you need to very seriously look into your dietary behaviour and prepare yourself for making significant changes on an ongoing basis.

Yo-Yo Dieting. Much has been discussed about yo-yo dieting in recent years. People often gain weight during religious festivals or while celebrating big occasions in the family. Then they feel guilty and start dieting and lose weight. Yet they gain back the lost weight at the next holiday season. Many of these people put themselves on lifelong dieting yet they never seem to lose weight. This type of yo-yo dieting is considered to be metabolically harmful.

As you already know, poor eating habits are usually responsible for being overweight. Most people in their middle years gain an excessive amount of weight. For successful weight loss, any type of crash diet or radical step followed for a short period of time is bound to fail. The extra weight is likely to come back unless you are prepared to commit yourself to a sensible lifelong approach to healthy eating habits.

Dietary Changes are a Must

Scientists have tried to study the role of dietary changes in the control of hypertension. Several studies have confirmed the benefits of a healthy diet. These studies have conclusively established that a diet rich in fruits, whole grains and low fat, lean meats and poultry not only helps in living longer but also by avoiding a diet high in saturated fat, you substantially cut down the risk of heart disease.

In a recent report[1] published in the journal *Circulation*, Dr Lawrence Appel from Johns Hopkins Medical School, has pointed out the benefit of a dietary approach to stop hypertension (DASH). This diet consists of low fat but high fruit and vegetable intake and has been noted to reduce blood pressure. The DASH diet has also been noted to lower the blood level of homocysteine (amino acid). High homocysteine levels have been implicated in causing coronary heart disease. Thus, if you are taking a DASH type of diet (low fat and high fruits and vegetables), then you are not only helping to reduce your blood pressure but also lowering your overall risk of heart disease because of a reduced blood homocysteine level.

If some people may find it harder to lose weight than others, it should be blamed on the genes. Neither is giving up the answer. Despite initial hurdles, most people who comply with a regular regimen of diet and exercise are successful in losing weight in the long run.

Role of Special Diets in Lowering Blood Pressure

Studies have been conducted to evaluate the role of special diets in lowering blood pressure. The DASH Study has been a topic of great interest. The effect on blood pressure with dietary changes was studied in detail by the scientists. Many of the following dietary changes were a part of the Dash Study.

- Reduced fat especially saturated fat.
- Low fat milk.
- Increased consumption of fruits.
- Increased intake of vegetables.
- Decreased intake of meat.
- Low consumption of refined sugar.
- Low intake of salt.
- Increased intake of fibre.

The positive effects of the dietary changes was first presented in the annual meeting of the American Heart Association in New Orleans in November 1996. Four hundred and fifty-nine adults at six different medical centres were included and subdivided into three different groups. One group was allowed to continue with the customary high fat diet, the second group was asked to consume a diet high in fruits and vegetables, and the third group was started on a combined low fat/low cholesterol and high fruits/vegetable diet. Interestingly, patients on the combined diet had the best results as far as their blood pressure was concerned. The best response in blood pressure reduction was noted in this third group. Patients on a high fruit and vegetable diet were asked to take an average of 8 to 10 servings of fruits and vegetables.

Although further studies should help to better understand the role of dietary changes, it is becoming clear that a low fat/low cholesterol vegetarian diet can help to lower blood pressure.

Role of Fish Oil

The role of fish oil in health promotion has been a matter of great interest for over 50 years. It has been noted that a special type of fish oil containing a high amount of omega-3 polyunsaturated fatty acids (n-3-PUFA) is helpful in reducing blood pressure. An intake of 3 to 6 gram of fish oil per day has been reported to lower blood pressure between 2 and 4 mmHg.

Most experts now believe that fish is good for the heart and cardiovascular system. In September 2000, for the first time, the American Heart Association, in its dietary recommendation stated that all adults should try to take at least two 3-ounce servings of fish a week. The results of an interesting study showing the benefits of fish intake were published in 1999 in *The Lancet*. Conducted by Indian physicians on 11,000 heart patients. Patients on a fish diet reduced their risk of dying from a second heart attack by approximately 17 per cent.

Fish oil has also been found to help in lowering cholesterol, thus reducing the risk of heart disease. It is recommended that if you have no particular reason to avoid fish in your diet, try to incorporate it at least 3 to 5 times a week for better cardiovascular function.

Role of Carbohydrates and Sugar

In a normal diet, 50-60 per cent of daily calories are provided by carbohydrates. Should patients with hypertension try to change this percentage? Dietary experiments with varying amounts of carbohydrate intake have been performed both in persons with normal blood pressure as well as in people with hypertension. Although no significant differences have been noted, excessive intake of refined sugar found to be associated with high blood pressure. Similarly, a high carbohydrate diet tends to raise insulin levels and may, therefore, interfere with weight reduction. In general, if you are hypertensive, try to lower your intake of refined sugar and carbohydrates.

Excessive consumption of sugar and sugar sweetened soft drinks not only contribute to obesity but also increase the risk of diabetes mellitus. It is estimated that the per capita consumption of sugar in the United States has gone up by 25 to 30 per cent in the past 15 years. No wonder that, we are witnessing a rapid rise in the incidence of obesity, hypertension and heart disease.

Role of Proteins

A normal adult diet probably includes 40 to 60 grams of protein per day. While in the Western world an average person tends to consume an excessive amount of protein, in the developing countries, protein intake tends to be somewhat low. In fact, protein calorie malnutrition is one of the most common forms of malnutrition in the developing world.

Some Foods Low in Carbohydrates

Foods	*Carb(g)*	*Foods*	*Carb(g)*
Apples	13.4	Lemon (sour lime)	8.0
Apricots (fresh)	11.6	Lemon (sweet)	7.3
Barley	19.6	Lettuce leaves	2.5
Bhekti (*Khajura*)	2.0	Lichees	14.0
Bittergourd	4.2	Melon (water)	3.3
Black Pomfret	2.0	Oatmeal	63.0
Bread (brown)	50.0	Orange juice	2.0
Brinjal	4.0	Orange	10.9
Butter milk	0.5	Papaya (ripe)	7.2
Cabbage	5.0	Peaches	10.5
Cauliflower	4.0	Pears	11.9
Coconut (tender)	6.0	Pineapple	10.8
Cucumber	2.5	Plums (red)	11.1
Curds	3.0	Pomegranate	14.5
Dates (fresh)	34.0	Pomfret	2.0
Drumstick	3.7	Radish (white)	3.4
Figs	7.6	Sole	2.2
French-beans	4.5	Soya beans	21.0
Grapes (green variety)	16.5	Spinach	3.0
Green gram (Mung)	57.0	Strawberries	10.0
Guava (country)	11.2	Tomato juice	4.1
Ladies Fingers	6.4	Tomatoes (fresh)	3.6
Leeks	17.2	Wheat germ	53.3

A diet high in protein (such as meat) is usually high in the acid load including hydrochloric, sulfuric and phosphoric acids. With so much acid intake, the kidneys have to work harder to get rid of these toxic acids and the associated waste products (ammonia generated from the breakdown of amino acids contained in the proteins). Both too little or too much protein in your diet can be a health hazard. While too little can cause muscle and body weakness, too much protein can impair kidney functions and cause high blood pressure in the long run. If your kidneys have been adversely affected by years of high blood pressure or if the high blood pressure has resulted because of the kidney disease itself, then it is important for you to discuss your total protein intake with your doctor.

Role of Fat

Almost everybody knows, or should know, that excessive fat in the diet is bad for heart. There are 9 calories in 1 gram of fat; protein and carbohydrates have 4.5 calories per gram. So the same weight of fat is going to make you fatter just because of the excessive calorie content. Diets low in fat, particularly saturated fat, have shown to help in the reduction of blood pressure. High fat intake is also a leading cause of heart disease. Remember, polyunsaturated fats are found in plants and are far more beneficial than saturated (animal) fats.

There are basically two types of polyunsaturated fats: omega 6 and omega 3 containing fatty acids. Omega 3 is found in fish and fish oils and omega 6 is found in vegetable oils (corn and soy bean oils). Replacing saturated fats with polyunsaturated fats is considered to be helpful for the heart. Hydrogenated vegetable oils (margarines) contain trans fatty acids and are harmful for the heart. Like saturated fats, margarine increases the total and LDL (bad) cholesterol and lowers the HDL (good) cholesterol.

The American Heart Association recommends that fat should provide no more than 30 per cent of daily calories. However, Dean Ornish, a world renowned cardiologist has argued that for the prevention of heart disease, you must lower your fat intake to less than 10 per cent as a source of total calories. Keeping your total fat intake as low as possible is certainly good for your blood pressure and your heart.

Role of Dietary Supplements in Lowering Blood Pressure

Over the years scientists have been interested in defining the role of calcium, potassium and magnesium supplements in the prevention and treatment of hypertension. Do these supplements really help to lower high blood pressure? Let us look at some of these issues.

Calcium Supplements. Low calcium intake has been known to be associated with high blood pressure. However, the benefits of calcium supplements or increasing the calcium intake in the diet for lowering of blood pressure has not been clearly established.

At the current time, most physicians generally do not prescribe calcium supplements for treatment of hypertension. However, there are two important facts to remember: firstly, ensuring the recommended daily allowance of 800 to 1500 mg of calcium per day in your diet is important, and secondly, it is advisable to discuss your daily diet with your doctor or dietitian to find the right answer. For a normal healthy adult calcium supplements are practically free from all side effects. However, for those who have high

Foods Rich in Calcium

- Milk and milk products
- Leafy vegetables
- Grapes
- Figs
- Watermelon
- Yogurt

blood pressure, taking an extra pill of calcium may require a discussion with the doctor.

Potassium Supplements. The relationship between potassium intake and blood pressure continues to be a matter of research. It is known that there is an inverse relationship between potassium intake and blood pressure levels. If potassium intake is low, the blood pressure readings tend to be higher and vice versa.

Foods Rich in Potassium

- Fresh fruits (banana, orange, etc)
- Milk
- Garlic
- Potato
- Radish

Studies involving potassium supplements have been conducted in both people with normal and with high blood pressure. In patients with lower blood (serum) potassium levels, potassium supplements have a significant impact of lowering the blood pressure. However, in an otherwise healthy person with a normal blood potassium level, the effect of potassium supplements tends to be very small. Altogether, for a normal person, taking extra potassium supplements is not considered to be a part of standard treatment for hypertension.

Potassium supplements are not altogether free from complications. In patients with poor kidney functions (especially patients with hypertension), unsupervised potassium supplement intake can lead to serious and potentially dangerous problems.

Magnesium Supplements. Magnesium deficiency has been linked to increased risk of hypertension, heart disease and osteoporosis. Magnesium is required to maintain the proper functioning of the smooth muscle wall of the arteries. While it is recommended that all adults take between 320 and 420 mg of magnesium per day, most people fail to consume over 200 mg per day.

Although the role of calcium, potassium and magnesium supplements still remains controversial, there are two specific situations to consider:

Foods Rich in Magnesium

❑ Beans	❑ Rice
❑ Almonds	❑ Spinach
❑ Lentils	❑ Baked potato
❑ Peanuts	❑ Yogurt
❑ Banana	❑ Peas
❑ Watermelon	❑ Grapefruit

1. If you are taking diuretics for the control of hypertension, you have a high risk of electrolyte disturbance (altered level of calcium, potassium and/or magnesium). If a particular deficiency is confirmed, you will need to take that particular supplement.

2. As a part of their general well being, many adults are routinely taking multivitamin tablets. Most of these pills have a small amount of calcium, potassium and magnesium. The use of multivitamins is considered to be fine for all adults. However, if you suffer from a kidney problem, you must discuss the use of these pills with your doctor since one or more of these supplements can interfere with your kidney functions, especially if you have high blood pressure.

References

1. Sacks Fm, Svetky LP, Vollmer WM, Appel LJ, Bray GA, Harsha D, Obarzanek E, Conlin PR, Miller ER 3rd, Simons-Morton DG, Karanja N, Lin PH. Summary of the scientific conference on dietary fatty acids and cardiovascular health: conference summary from the nutrition committee of the American Heart Association. Circulation. 2001 Feb 20; 103 (7): 1034-9.

17

Treating Hypertension with Drugs

Poisons and medicine are often times the same substance given with different intents.

Peter Mere Latham
1789-1875

The world has changed in the last few decades. Medical science has made rapid and breakthrough progress. There is a much better understanding of the causes, effects and complications of hypertension. Several major classes of drugs have been developed. Longer acting drugs have made a big difference; these medicines do not need to be taken more than once a day.

With the increasing number of medications available to treat hypertension, medical scientists have been focussing more on the effectiveness and problems associated with each individual group of medications.

Major groups of medication for treatment of hypertension are:

- Diuretics

- Centrally Acting Drugs
- Alpha-Adrenergic Receptor Blockers
- Beta Receptor Blockers
- Direct Vasodilators
- Indirect Vasodilators
- Angiotensin II Receptor Blockers (ARBs)

Diuretics

It is interesting to note that even though diuretics have been in use for over 40 years, their precise mode of action in reducing blood pressure remains unclear. Besides the treatment of hypertension, diuretics are also widely used to treat congestive heart failure and other conditions associated with collection of fluid in the body.

Basically, a diuretic type of drug works by increasing the volume of urine excreted from the body. The first significant diuretic, chlorothiazide, became available in 1957 and was soon followed by hydrochlorothiazide in 1958.

Even though the use of diuretics has declined in the recent past, the US Joint National Committee on Detection, Evaluation and Treatment of High Blood Pressure[1] continues to strongly recommend the use of diuretics and/or beta blockers as the first line of drug treatment for uncomplicated hypertension. In fact, no other group of anti-hypertensive medications has been tested and found to be as effective as diuretics in the reduction of morbidity and mortality.

For treatment of hypertension in the elderly, diuretics are generally accepted to be far more effective than beta blockers as first line therapy.

Within the kidney, different diuretics work in different ways. While the precise mechanism of action of various diuretics is best left to the understanding of your physician, it is only appropriate that you familiarise yourself with some of the commonly used names in the diuretic category.

Thiazide Diuretics. These are most frequently used class of diuretics. In most cases the doctor will prescribe one of the thiazide diuretics for the control of hypertension.

Drugs	*Usual Daily Dose*
Benzthiazide	12.5-50 mg
Cholorthiazide	125-500 mg
Hydrochlorothiazide	12.5-50 mg
Polythiazide	1-4 mg
Chlorothalidone (hygroton)	12.5-50 mg
Metolazone	0.5-1 mg

The thiazide diuretics inhibit and interfere with sodium and chloride absorption in the kidney tubules and thus a lot of water and electrolytes are excreted from the body. With the reduced fluid volume, the cardiac volume goes down and that results in lowering blood pressure. However, this diuretic effect is noted to be most effective only in the first few weeks. Studies have indicated that the fluid volume returns to its original baseline after a few weeks of treatment with diuretics.

Is your blood pressure adequately controlled with your current dose of thiazide diuretic? The current recommendations by hypertension experts would suggest that since very high doses of a single agent are usually associated with side effects, it may be a better idea to add another drug from another group (ACE inhibitor or betablocker, for example) for better control of hypertension.

Loop Diuretics. While thiazide diuretics are most commonly used for the control of hypertension, it is important to know a little bit about the loop diuretics as well.

Loop diuretics are far more potent and have a rapid onset of action but have a shorter duration of action. These are powerful diuretics but are less commonly used for the control of hypertension unless the blood pressure is severely high. Loop diuretics are far more commonly used for congestive heart failure.

Drugs	*Usual Daily Dose*
Bumetanide	0.5-5mg
Furosemide	20-240mg
Ethacrynic acid	25-100mg

The most commonly used loop diuretics is furosemide (LASIX). A comparatively new loop diuretic is bumetinide (BUMEX) which is up to forty times more potent than LASIX. However, both LASIX and BUMEX are not the diuretic of first choice in the treatment of hypertension and are mostly reserved for the use of conditions like congestive heart failure.

Diuretics have been recently compared with alpha blockers in the Antihypertensive and Lipid Lowering to Prevent Heart Attacks Trial (ALLHAT trial)[2]. In this study, compared to diuretics, patients on alpha blockers were noted to have 25 per cent more complications and twice as likely to be admitted to the hospital with congestive heart failure. Diuretics were judged to be far more safe and superior to alpha blockers in the treatment of hypertension.

Thiazide and Loop Diuretics: Side Effects

Side Effects	Test		Treatment
Low Sodium	Irritability, confusion, dryness of tongue and skin, loss of elasticity of skin, sunken eyes.	Blood test (normal level 136-145 meq/L)	Decrease or stop diuretics, treat with other agents.
High Blood Sugar	Passing excessive urine (polyuria), excessive thirst (polydipsia), excessive appetitie (polyphasia), increased infections.	Blood sugar level	Decrease or discontinue diuretic, may require increasing dose of diabetic pill or insulin.
High Cholesterol	No symptoms	Blood test	Stop or reduce diuretics, dietary changes, may require medications to control cholesterol.
High Uric Acid	Acute, painful, swelling of the joint (most commonly the big toe)	Blood test	Decrease or discontinue diuretic, use other choices, may need treatment for gout/high uric acid.
High Calcium	Disturbed appetite, constipation, nausea and vomiting	Blood test	Discontinue or decrease diuretic, consider other choices, increase fluid intake.

Potassium Sparing Diuretics. There are two important facts to remember about potassium sparing diuretics. Firstly, on their own, they are only weak diuretics and therefore, need to be given with thiazide or loop diuretics for better effectiveness. Secondly, since these diuretics prevent the loss of potassium in the urine and thus may raise blood (serum) potassium levels, they should be used with caution in patients with poor kidney function. High potassium levels can cause serious problems with the proper functioning of the heart.

Drugs	*Usual Daily Dose*
Amiloride	5-10 mg
Spironolactone	25-100 mg
Triameterine	50-150 mg

Again, potassium sparing diuretics are not commonly used for hypertension treatment but are considered to be very good choices for the treatment of conditions like congestive heart failure.

Toxicity and Side Effects of Diuretics. It may be safe to state that no drug is completely safe and free from side effects. All three types of diuretics (thiazide, loop, potassium sparing) have their own side effects.

Drugs	*Side Effects*
Thiazide and Loop diuretics	Low sodium level Low potassium level High calcium level High uric acid High blood sugar High cholesterol Sexual dysfunction
Potassium sparing diuretics	High potassium level Gynaecomastia (due to spironolactone)

Some of the side effects are, indeed, serious. For example, if significantly low levels of potassium develop due to prolonged diuretic use, the risk of death due to sudden cardiac irregularities is far higher as compared to a patient with normal potassium levels in the blood. Additionally, for someone with left ventricular hypertrophy due to hypertension, low potassium level becomes increasingly a serious risk factor. Unfortunately it is not always easy or practical to have a lifelong daily or even a weekly blood test for the measurement of sodium, potassium or blood sugar just because a person is taking a diuretic.

What, then, is the best way to recognise the side effects or even prevent some of the problems associated with diuretic use. Since low potassium is a normal accompaniment of thiazide or loop diuretic treatment, it is a common practice to prescribe supplemental potassium.

Despite the side effects listed above, diuretics remain a major choice of drugs for the treatment of hypertension. Fortunately, the incidence of serious complications remains very low. Besides being very effective in controlling blood pressure, diuretics are perhaps the least expensive group of medication.

Centrally Acting Drugs

Drugs that primarily work because of their central action have been available for many years. The most commonly used centrally acting agents are:

- Methyl-dopa (Aldomet)
- Clonidine
- Reserpine

In the last few decades due to the availability of better and safer alternative choices, the use of centrally acting agents has declined considerably. Not surprisingly, the US Joint National Committee on Hypertension in its report did not favour the use of these medications as their first choice.

Let us look at some of these medications in a little more detail:

Methyl-Dopa. Methyl-dopa or Aldomet has been available for over forty years. Before beta blockers became widely available, Methyl-dopa was used as a major group of drugs (with or without diuretics) for the treatment of hypertension.

Side effects

- Weight gain/fluid retention
- Sedation and drowsiness
- Depression
- Nasal stuffiness
- Sexual impotence
- Liver damage
- Unexplained fever
- Haemolytic anaemia
- Postural hypotension
- Lupus like syndrome

Clonidine. Clonidine is a powerful antihypertensive agent. Clonidine works by controlling nerve impulses and helps in the relaxation of blood vessels so that blood passes through them more easily. This helps to lower blood pressure.

However, because of availability of better drugs, clonidine is not considered to be the first choice of drugs in the management of hypertension.

Side effects

- Dry mouth
- Drowsiness and sedation
- Depression (do not take clonidine if you are on tricyclic antidepressant drugs like imipramine)

Reserpine. Reserpine was the earliest drug that was developed from Rauwolfia alkaloid grown in the foothills of the Himalayas. Newer and much better agents are now available. Reserpine tends to be a less potent medication.

Side effects

- Nasal stuffiness.
- Depression.
- Gastrointestinal upset.
- Weight gain.
- Breast cancer.
- Risk of depression and cancer.

Alpha-Adrenergic Receptor Blockers

Alpha-adrenergic receptor blockers are a separate class of medication that have been used in the treatment of hypertension for many years. However, as compared to the other group of drugs, only a small percentage of patients are noted to be taking alpha-blockers. Why so?

First the US Joint National Committee of experts on hypertension continues to favour drugs like diuretics and beta receptor blockers primarily because of their long proven track record and safety in the treatment of hypertension. Second, calcium channel blockers and ACE Inhibitors have also been widely used because of their potency and efficacy in reducing blood pressure.

There are three important drugs within the class of alpha-blockers that are in common use and these are

Alpha blockers	*Usual Daily Dose*
Prozosin (Minipress)	1-20 mg three times a day
Terazosin (Hytrin)	1-20 mg twice a day
Doxazosin (Cardura)	1-16 mg once a day

Let us, first of all, look at some of the benefits of alpha-blockers.

Alpha-blockers are especially helpful in hypertensive patients with co-existing problems of benign prostatic hypertrophy (BPH). Prostate is a walnut size structure located below the urinary bladder and is an important gland for normal sexual function in men. After the age of 50, because of hormonal changes, this gland starts increasing in size (hypertrophy) and causing problems in urination (frequency and urgency of urination are common symptoms). Over 40 per cent of men over the age of 50 are found to develop BPH. Alpha-blockers are particularly helpful in relieving the symptoms of BPH, and are commonly recommended for hypertensive patients with BPH.

Another advantage of alpha-blockers is that they have no effect on lipids (blood cholesterol) and blood sugar whereas drugs like diuretics and beta receptor blockers adversely effect blood sugar as well as lipids. Hypertensive patients with the problem of high cholesterol or high blood sugar (diabetes mellitus), are a good candidate for alpha-blockers.

It is estimated that currently between 2-4 per cent of all hypertensive patients are being prescribed alpha-blockers in the United States.

Beta Receptor Blockers

Beta receptor blockers were first developed or discovered in England by Dr Black, who received Nobel prize for his wonderful work. Because of the proven track record of success with beta receptor blockers in numerous large scale scientific studies, beta receptor blockers have received constant praise and a seal of approval from most scientific organisations and world renowned experts in hypertension. For more than 20 years, the American Joint National Committee on Hypertension has consistently recommended the use of beta receptor blockers as its first choice.

Beta receptor blockers should be considered to be very effective and generally a safe choice for treatment of hypertension in the vast majority of patients.

Currently there are over two dozen choices within the group of beta receptor blockers. Cardioselectivity is one of the important characteristics of beta blockers. This means that the drug is primarily working on the heart and will have less side effects like bronchospasm. Acebutalol, Atenolol and Metoprolol have better cardioselectivity and are, therefore, preferable to other beta blockers. This consideration is more important in patients with asthma and chronic obstructive pulmonary disease (bronchitis or emphysema).

Beta Receptor Blockers: Some Advantages

- Generally safe, with a proven record of reducing mortality and morbidity.
- Beta blockers reduce cardiac output and are therefore specially helpful in patients with increased cardiac output (hyperkinetic hypertension).
- Specially helpful in hypertension patients who have high anxiety, stress and migraine.
- Useful for hypertensive patients with co-existing diseases such as cardiac arrhythmias, angina

pectoris, cardiomyopathy and congestive heart failure.

- Helpful for patients who have already had a heart attack since beta receptor blockers may prevent a second heart attack and sudden death.
- Maybe safely used with other antihypertensive agents.
- Reduce heart rate and contractility.
- Reduce peripheral vascular resistance.

Some of the beta blockers and their dose frequencies are listed below.

Beta blockers	*Usual Daily Dose*
Acebutolol *(Sectral)*	200 mg twice daily
Atenolol *(Tenormin)*	25-100 mg daily
Pindalol *(Visken)*	5 mg twice daily
Penbutolol *(Levatol)*	20 mg daily
Metoprolol *(Lopressor)*	100 mg daily
Propranolol *(Inderal)*	10-30 mg 2-4 times daily
Propranolol Long Acting *(Inderal LA)*	80-320 mg daily
Nadolol	40-300 mg daily
Bisoprolol	2.5 mg daily
Pindolol	5-15 mg twice daily
Carvedolol	3.125-25 mg twice daily
Labetalol	100-400 mg twice daily
Timolol	20-60 mg twice daily

Trade names may vary in different countries.

Although somewhat less important, lipid solubility of a beta-blocker is also considered as an important factor in the selection of a beta-blocker.

In general, it is better to take a beta-blocker that is cardioselective and is water soluble (as compared to fat soluble). Cardioselective beta receptor blockers also tend to cause less lipid disturbances. Moreover, for someone who happens to be diabetic and suffers from hypertension, a beta-1 selective beta-blocker is advised.

High lipid solubility beta receptor blockers are far more commonly associated with neuropsychiatric symptoms like sleep difficulties, increased dreaming, difficulty in concentration and higher incidence of nervousness.

Common examples of low lipid soluble beta receptor blockers include acebutolol and atenolol.

Do non-selective beta receptor blockers such as timolol and bisoprolol offer any advantages? Yes, but only in conditions other than cardiovascular problems. In patients with migraine and tremor, non selective beta receptor blockers have been noted to be more effective than beta-1 cardioselective agents.

Side Effects of Beta Receptor Blockers. Like all other medications, beta receptor blockers too have side effects. As mentioned earlier, non-selective beta receptor blockers and beta receptor blockers with a high degree of lipid solubility tend to have far more serious side effects as compared to the beta-1 cardioselective agents and water soluble beta receptor blockers. Major side effects of beta receptor blockers are as below:

Effects on Nervous System. Sleep disturbance, sadness bad dreams (nightmares), hallucinations and confusion are some of the side effects that are more commonly seen with lipid soluble (Propranolol and Metoprolol) agents.

Although in early studies, there were reports of depression being caused by beta receptor blockers, the incidence of depression with beta receptor blockers is not very high.

Interference with Diabetes Mellitus. A particular risk of complication of beta-blocker therapy must be understood by those with diabetes and taking insulin or any other medicine to control blood sugar. All diabetic patients are at risk of experiencing low blood sugar (hypoglycemia), particularly if they happen to miss their meals or take excessive anti-diabetic tablets or insulin.

Beta receptor blockers interfere with body's response to elevate the blood sugar if there is a low blood sugar (hypoglycemic) episode. Beta receptor blockers also tend to increase insulin resistance. Fortunately, this risk is only a small one. It is important for everyone taking beta receptor blockers whether diabetic or not to get blood sugar checked at least once a year.

Lipid Problems with Beta Receptor Blockers. Beta receptor blockers may upset lipid profile. One or more of the following problems may be associated with the intake of beta receptor blockers — high total cholesterol, high LDL (bad cholesterol), high triglyceride and/or low HDL (good cholesterol).

In general, beta receptor blockers that are cardioselective have minimal effects on lipid levels.

Excessive Tiredness. The problem of excessive fatigue and tiredness is often/sometimes initially experienced by those starting on beta receptor blockers. Fortunately, in most people, after a few weeks the sense of tiredness tends to improve and they are able to perform normal daily routine despite taking tablets.

If you think that you are not even able to carry on with your daily activities while being on beta receptor blockers, then you need to discuss the problem with your doctor.

Sexual Impotence. Sexual impotence is a recognised side effect of beta receptor blockers. While some patients may benefit by switching to another brand of beta receptor blocker, others may have to switch to another class of medication. If you experience such problems you need to discuss these thoroughly with your physician.

Combined Alpha and Beta Receptor Blockers. This is a separate class of medication that has both alpha and beta blocking properties. The two best known examples are Labetalol and Carvedolol. Labetalol has alpha and beta blocking potency in the ratio of 1:4. Both Labetalol and Carvedolol are known selective beta receptor blockers. In general, these drugs result in the reduction of peripheral vascular resistance and thus cause a fall in the blood pressure. Labetalol has been mainly used for emergency treatment of hypertension, hypertension during pregnancy and in patients with poor kidney functions. Since other better agents are available for control of hypertension, Labetalol is not considered to be a preferred choice for general use in the management of hypertension. Carvedolol has recently received a lot more attention since it has been noted to significantly reduce the mortality in patients with congestive heart failure. Headaches, dizziness, scalp itching, liver damage and excessive fall in the blood pressure are some of the side effects.

Direct Vasodilators

Vasodilators are drugs that directly enter the wall of the blood vessels and cause them to dilate and relax, resulting in lower blood pressure. Drugs that are commonly included in the group of vasodilators are as below.

- Hydralazine
- Nitroprusside
- Nitroglycerin
- Minoxidil
- Diazoxide

Direct vasodilators are currently considered to be only a third line of choice of drugs for the routine control of hypertension (diuretics, beta-blockers, ACE Inhibitors and calcium channel blockers are better choices). In selected situations, however, Hydralazine may have to be used and these situations specifically include hypertension with kidney damage, severe resistant hypertension and/or hypertensive emergencies.

The usual doses and side effects of the commonly used vasodilators are listed in the table. One of the serious side effects like lupus syndrome can only be diagnosed by your doctor. Fever, facial rashes are the hallmark of lupus-like syndrome. It is fortunately not a very common side effect of these drugs.

Commonly used Vasodilators

Vasodilators	*Usual Daily Dose*	*Side Effects/Comments*
Hydralazine	25 mg thrice daily	Headaches, increased heart rate, flushing, lupus like syndrome, nausea and vomiting, muscle cramps, diarrhoea
Minoxidil	2.5-10 mg daily	Excessive hair growth (hirsutism), pericardial effusion,fluid retention and edema

Indirect Vasodilators

Indirect vasodilators work indirectly on the walls of the blood vessels to prevent them from contracting. The drugs in this group are :

- Calcium channel blockers
- ACE Inhibitors
- Alpha blockers

Calcium Channel Blockers. In recent years calcium channel blockers or calcium antagonists have become one of the major class of drugs for the treatment of hypertension. Besides high blood pressure, calcium channel blockers are also widely used for coronary artery disease.

In simple terms, calcium blockers inhibit the flow of calcium through numerous calcium channels. With this blockage, the smooth muscles of the blood vessels become relaxed and widened. This leads to lower peripheral vascular resistance and to lower blood pressure. Although the blood pressure lowering effect of calcium blockers is mainly achieved because of relaxation of the blood vessels, these drugs are also thought to lower the blood pressure through their beneficial effects on the kidneys and hormones in the body.

Preferred use for Calcium Channel Blockers. Calcium channel blockers are especially useful in the following situations:

1. Hypertension with atrial tachycardia or atrial fibrillation.
2. Hypertension with angina.
3. Hypertension with diabetes mellitus.
4. Hypertension with migraine.

Calcium channel blockers may also have drug to drug interactions. Because of the risk of side effects, if you are taking one or more of the following medications, you must discuss the concurrent use of calcium channel blockers with your doctor:

- Digoxin
- Quinidine
- Dilantin
- Propranolol
- Prazosin
- Theophylline
- Rifampin

What is Good about Calcium Channel Blockers? The safety profile of calcium channel blockers is generally good and are useful for men and women, and for patients of all ages.

They are as effective as beta blockers, diuretics or ACE Inhibitors in controlling blood pressure. If used as monotherapy, will successfully bring the blood pressure within normal range in up to 50 per cent of patients.

Specifically, calcium channel blockers are effective in the treatment of left ventricular hypertrophy and useful for patients with coronary heart disease and cardiac arrhythmias.

There are no contraindication in use for patients with high blood pressure and associated peripheral vascular disease or bronchial asthma. There are no adverse effects on lipids (unlike beta blockers or diuretics), blood sugar (unlike beta blockers or diuretics) or on electrolytes (unlike beta blockers or diuretics).

The following are commonly used calcium channel blockers

- Nifedipine (PROCARDIA)
- Verapamil (CALAN, ISOPTIN)
- Diltiazem (CARDIZEM)

- Nicardipine (CARDENE)
- Amlodipine (NORVASC)
- Felodipine (PLENDIL)
- Isradipine (DYNACIRC)

Ace Inhibitors. As compared to the early days of treatment of hypertension, we are now fortunate to have a number of alternative choices. In recent years, this choice has been significantly widened with the availability of drugs that are called Angiotensin Converting Enzyme (ACE) inhibitors. Although the search for the ideal antihypertensive agent still continues, Ace Inhibitors have become a major class of drugs for the treatment of hypertension mainly because of their beneficial properties.

In the highly acclaimed HOPE trial (Heart Outcomes Prevention Evaluation), treatment with ACE Inhibitor (Ramipril)[2] was reported to cut the risk of cardiovascular deaths, heart attacks and strokes by 22 per cent. Dr Salim Yusuf, Professor of Medicine, McMaster University, Hamilton, Ontario, Canada, was the chief investigator of the HOPE trial that involved patients over the age of 55 with a history of coronary heart disease, peripheral vascular disease, stroke, or patients who had diabetes mellitus or one or more coronary risk factors. This study clearly demonstrated the significant benefits of the ACE Inhibitor type of medication.

Altogether, the net effect and advantages of ACE Inhibitors are as below.

1. Peripheral vascular resistance is lowered.
2. Heart rate, cardiac output remains unaffected.

3. Left ventricular hypertrophy is reversed.
4. Kidney functions are improved.
5. In patients with heart failure, ACE Inhibitors are noted to lower morbidity as well as mortality.
6. There are no adverse effects on electrolytes, and blood lipid levels.
7. ACE Inhibitors may be safely used with most other drugs including diuretics and beta blockers.
8. The overall quality of life is noted to be better with the use of ACE Inhibitors as compared to other medications.

For cases of diabetes mellitus with hypertension, and of congestive heart failure with hypertension, ACE Inhibitors are recommended as the first choice.

You might ask that if Ace Inhibitors are so good, why are these drugs not the first choice for all hypertension patients. The reasons are clear. It is only because we have a number of proven studies with diuretics and beta blockers showing their efficacy in reducing the death rate over the past 30 years. In view of such strong evidence, diuretics and beta blockers still remain the first line treatment. As yet, we do not have concrete studies confirming the long-term effects and benefits of ace inhibitors.

Angiotensin II Receptor Blockers (ARBs)

In the past ten years, a new class of drugs called Angiotensin II Receptor Blockers (ARBs) have been developed. It has been noted that there are two types of receptors in the body: angiotensin receptor ATI and ATII. It is the ATI receptor that is most actively involved in the contraction of blood vessels and the heart. Losartan has become one of the most widely used angiotensin II receptor blocker drugs in the treatment of hypertension. Because of the increasing success of drugs from this group, other medications, including Valsartan and Irbesartan, have also been introduced in the market in the past three years. By attaching to the ATI receptors, these medications neutralise the effects of angiotensin II in the body. Once again, it is important to note that, while with the ACE Inhibitors the levels of angiotensin II would be reduced, with the use of ARBs, the level of angiotensin II in the blood remains high. However, if the receptors where angiotensin II could have worked are already blocked by ARBs, the high amount of circulating angiotensin II cannot cause any harm. On the other hand, because of the ATI receptors being blocked, there is a desirable fall in the blood pressure.

Side effects

- Dry cough.
- Mild rise in potassium levels.
- Oedema of the legs.
- Taste disturbance.
- Skin rashes.

Are ARB type of drugs as effective as other types of medications in lowering blood pressure? The short answer is probably, yes. Losartan, one of the earliest ARB type of drugs, has been compared to several other groups of medications for its efficacy in the treatment of hypertension. Losartan, 50 mg per day, and Enalapril, (an ACE Inhibitor) 5-10 mg per day have been reported to have similar effects in lowering blood pressure. Losartan has also been compared to Amlodipine, a calcium channel blocker. Once again, the effectiveness of Losartan has been noted to be similar to the effectiveness of calcium channel blockers. Besides being effective, the ARBs have so far been noted to be quite safe with few side effects.

In the United States and Europe, several ARBs are now available. In fact, many physicians are choosing ARBs over ACE Inhibitors as their first choice. The expert committees on hypertension have so far recommended that ARBs should be used only if you are not able to tolerate the usual ACE Inhibitor type of drugs for the control of hypertension.

One of the major side effects of ACE Inhibitors is chronic dry cough in up to ten per cent of patients. If you happen to be taking Ace Inhibitors and have no significant side effects, including dry cough, then perhaps there is no need to change from ACE Inhibitors to ARBs. In many ways, many of these ARBs are still being evaluated in different scientific studies.

Because there is a risk to the foetus, ACE Inhibitors must *not* be taken by pregnant women, especially during the second and third trimester.

References

1. Chobanian AV, Bakris GL, Black HR, Cushman WC, Green LA, Izzo JL Jr, Jones DW, Materson BJ, Oparil S, Wright JT Jr, Roccella EJ; Joint National Committee on Prevention, Detection, Evaluation and Treatment of High Blood Pressure. National Heart, Lung and Blood Institute; National High Blood Pressure Education Program Coordinating Committee. Seventh report of the Joint National Committee on Prevention, Detection, Evaluation and Treatment of High Blood Pressure. Boston University School of Medicine, Boston, Mass, USA. Hypertension. 2003 Dec; 42 (6): 1206-52.
2. Weinsaft JW, O'Rourke MF, Nichols WW, Sharma AM, Pischon T, Engeli S, Gavras H, Francis G. Effect of Ramipril on Cardiovascular Events in High-Risk Patients. N Engl J Med 2000; 343: 64-66, Jul 6, 2000

18

Step-Up Care and Combined Therapy

The mistake of all that medical talk lies in the very fact that it connects the idea of health with the idea of care. What has health to do with care? Health has to do with carelessness.

Gilbert Keith Chesterton
1905

Until a few years ago, physicians were typically taught during their medical school years that they must try to treat one disease with one drug alone and limit the use of multiple drugs for the treatment of a single disease. In many ways, this advice sounded very sensible. However, it is now believed that if only one drug is used for the treatment of hypertension, less than 50 per cent of patients can expect to have good control. If another drug is added to the treatment, the control of hypertension becomes possible in up to 80 per cent of patients. The addition of a third drug is noted to provide further help. With the use of three different types of drugs for the treatment of hypertension, blood pressure in over 90 per cent of patients can be controlled satisfactorily.

The above observations have made a huge impact on the prescribing habits and, indeed, became the basis for the step-up care type of approach in the treatment of hypertension. The step-up care approach works as below:

1. The physician first starts on the lowest dose of one antihypertensive agent — Drug A.

2. Depending upon the blood pressure response, the dose of Drug A is gradually increased by the doctor.

3. If the maximum dose of Drug A still fails to control blood pressure, the doctor adds Drug B to the treatment.

4. If now with Drug A and Drug B the blood pressure is controlled satisfactorily, then it is just fine. If the blood pressure is still high, despite using the maximum doses of Drug A and Drug B, the physician would then add Drug C to the treatment.

This step-up care approach has been used for over 25 years in clinical practice by physicians all over the world. Raising the dose of a particular drug, however, does not always have the expected effect in terms of lowering the blood pressure. It has been observed that beyond a stage any further dose increase does not have the same effect. Infact it may start having adverse impact on the health. For example, higher doses of the diuretics beyond a stage could result in serious side effects including electrolyte deficiencies (low sodium, potassium levels, etc.). Just like diuretics, other types of antihypertensive medications have also been noted to be most beneficial in lowering blood pressure when used in moderate and not in extremely high doses which may lead to undesirable side effects.

Combination Drug Therapy

In the last few years, combination drug therapy has become important. Our understanding of the value of combination therapy for the treatment of hypertension has improved significantly. Smaller doses of two drugs (combination therapy), have a much better chance of bringing blood pressure under control with very little risk of side effects. Since different antihypertensive medications have a different mode of action, combination therapy is considered to be the best way to treat most hypertension patients.

In one of the earliest scientific reports, Dr William Frishman, a world-renowned cardiologist and his colleagues had shown that even very low doses of a diuretic can potentiate the blood pressure reducing effect of another drug without causing adverse metabolic side effects. Their pioneering study was published in the *Archives of Internal Medicine* in 1994.

In a study by Dr Elliott and his colleagues published in the *American Journal of Hypertension* in July 1999, a combination of calcium channel blockers and Ace Inhibitors was found to be very helpful in controlling hypertension in over 85 per cent of patients. Similar results were presented by Dr Joel N. Neutel, Professor of Medicine at the University of California, at the 14th Scientific Meeting of the American Society of Hypertension held in New York City in May 1999.

Why does Combination Therapy work Better? Hypertension is a complex disease with several mechanisms that result in the rise of your blood pressure. Different drugs used for the treatment of hypertension work in a variety of ways to bring blood pressure under control. Unfortunately, as yet, there is no single ideal drug that can control blood pressure with no side effects. Combination treatment is helpful because a second drug can circumvent the physiological and/or pharmacological unwanted effect of the first drug. For example, beta blockers tend to cause salt and water retention and thus cause an increase in the body plasma volume. The addition of a small dose of a diuretic in a fixed dose combination therapy can help in controlling the extra body fluid and lowering the blood pressure.

Is combination therapy the treatment of choice for everybody with high blood pressure? Combination therapy is, of course, not required for someone who has stage I hypertension and has good control of his or her blood pressure with only one type of medication. In general, combination therapy is considered to be your best choice if:

1. Your blood pressure is significantly high (systolic blood pressure over 160 and diastolic blood pressure over 100).

2. If your blood pressure remains uncontrolled with the use of one type of drug alone (monotherapy).

3. If you are experiencing side effects with high doses of a single drug.

4. If you are over the age of 60, then your risk of developing drug side effects is much lower if you take low dose combination therapy.

The report from the US Joint National Committee on Hypertension has clearly favoured the approach of combining low doses of two agents from two different antihypertensive medication groups for a safer and more effective control of hypertension.

19

Step-Down Care

There are no really 'safe' biologically active drugs.
There are only 'safe' physicians.

Harold A. Kaminetzky
1963

It is generally accepted that once you are hypertensive you are always hypertensive. In other words, you need treatment for the rest of your life. In most cases, physicians as well as patients strongly believe that once you have been taking blood pressure medications for a few years you will perhaps never be able to do without the pills.

While it is true that hypertension requires life-long appropriate control in a small percentage of patients whose blood pressure has been under very good control with a gradual reduction of medications may be tried. Scientific studies have indicated that although in more than 95 per cent of patients, high blood pressure returns upon discontinuing medication, in less than 5 per cent of patients, the blood pressure may remain under control even without the medications.

This small group of patients who may continue to have normal blood pressure readings despite taking no drugs generally have the following characteristics:

1. They are usually younger patients.
2. They perhaps have high-normal or stage I type of hypertension.
3. They are now taking very little salt.
4. They are not drinking alcohol.
5. They are no longer overweight and have lost significant weight.

In most cases, such patients have been noted to have made significant lifestyle changes. Whatever the reasons, if you happen to be taking only a small dose of one type of medication (for example, Atenolol 25 mg) and over 95 per cent of your readings are within normal range, then you should discuss the possibility of discontinuing medication with your doctor. It is not advisable to discontinue the medication on your own.

In one study[1], over 90 per cent of mildly hypertensive patients remained free of high blood pressure after discontinuation of drugs when monitored over a period of four years.

The first step is to have a very careful assessment done by your doctor. Based on record of several blood pressure readings, your physician may decide to slowly cut down or stop medication altogether. How would you then know whether you can do without the medications or whether you will need to start taking the pills once again? Only regular blood pressure checks once or twice a week, over a period of many months can give the right answer. It's only a matter of trial. There is no magic trick to find out whether a person will need to restart the medication or not.

References

1. Schmieder RE, Rockstruth JK, Messerli FH. Antihypertensive Therapy. To Stop or Not to Stop? JAMA 1991, 265: 1566-1571.

20

Hypertension and Diabetes Mellitus

When a man loses his health, then he first begins to take care of it.

Josh Billings
1818-1885

Diabetes mellitus is a serious chronic disease and the incidence of diabetes mellitus is on the rise in almost all countries. In countries like India, increasing levels of affluence have lead to increase in obesity and adult onset (type 2) diabetes mellitus. Altogether, experts strongly believe that the number of people with diabetes mellitus will continue to rise all over the world for the foreseeable future.

As compared to non-diabetics, diabetic patients are

- two to four times more at risk of developing heart disease;
- two to three times more at risk of developing stroke; and
- two to three times more at risk of dying prematurely

Complications of Hypertension and Diabetes Mellitus

It is estimated that the risk of developing hypertension is doubled in those who have diabetes mellitus. Since both hypertension as well as diabetes have their own complications, the total risk of complications, such as coronary heart disease, increases substantially. In view of this seriousness, the US Joint National Committee on Hypertension has emphasised that for persons with diabetes and hypertension an ideal goal of blood pressure control is below 130/85 and not 140/90 mmHg. Unfortunately, only about 16 per cent of people with hypertension and diabetes mellitus are reported to have good blood pressure control. Keeping blood pressure below 140/90 is fine if the hypertension is uncomplicated, i.e., not associated with another disease like diabetes mellitus.

The fact that diabetes mellitus increases the risk of developing hypertension has been known for over fifty years. Diabetes mellitus causes changes in the small and large blood vessels of the heart and kidneys. In the presence of hypertension, these changes are further accelerated. Thus, a vicious cycle can get established, increasing the risk of developing many of the above complications. Diabetes mellitus remains a leading cause of end stage renal failure with millions of patients requiring kidney dialysis on a regular basis.

Risk of Kidney Failure. Scientific studies have now established that patients with poor control of diabetes mellitus are far more likely to develop kidney failure. In the famous United Kingdom Prospective Diabetic Study

(UKPDS)[1], tight blood pressure control was noted to be even more important and effective than blood glucose control in patients who had both diabetes mellitus and hypertension.

What is the significance of all this information? If you are a diabetic, it is important keep a record of your blood pressure. If your blood pressure is within normal range, then you do not require any medications. If blood pressure is found to be high, you need to take appropriate steps including medications to bring blood pressure below 130/80. In all cases, all diabetics must pay full attention and maintain a lifestyle that would help in controlling not only the diabetes mellitus but also the blood pressure.

Decrease in Mental Functions. Patients with diabetes mellitus and hypertension have also been reported to have a decline in their mental functions. In a study published in the Journal Neurology, Dr Knopman and his colleagues from the famous Mayo Clinic reported the result of 10,000 adults (ages 47 to 70 years) and noted that patients with hypertension and diabetes mellitus had a decline with the speed of doing things mentally. Healthy adults with neither disease had the best results, patients with one disease (hypertension or diabetes mellitus) faired worse and those with both conditions were noted to have the lowest score on mental function testing.

Selection of Medications

Should a diabetic and who has developed hypertension focus more on the control of diabetes mellitus or hypertension or both? The answer is simple. It is the control of both hypertension and diabetes mellitus that can save a person from long term complications of these two dreadful diseases.

ACE Inhibitors. A number of studies have confirmed that ACE Inhibitors are the drug of choice for diabetic patients with hypertension. This group of drugs (examples are Captopril and Enalapril), have few adverse metabolic effects and therefore do not interfere with the control of diabetes mellitus. Ace Inhibitors also result in slowing the progression of diabetic nephropathy and help in reducing urinary protein loss.

In the widely quoted HOPE study (Heart Outcomes Prevention Evaluation)[2] Ramipril (an ACE Inhibitor) not only successfully helped better blood pressure control but also contributed to an overall reduction in cardiovascular complications and death. The doctor must rule out the presence of renal artery stenosis, a rare condition characterised by the hardening and narrowing of the kidney arteries. In the presence of renal artery stenosis, Ace Inhibitors may cause serious complications including kidney failure. Frequent monitoring of electrolytes is also important for anyone taking Ace

> Lifestyle changes, including salt reduction, weight loss and regular physical exercise are likely to help in the control of both diabetes as well as hypertension. Even with or without the pills for hypertension, the importance of lifestyle modifications must not be underestimated. Some patients wrongly assume that by taking blood pressure medications, they need not bother too much about lifestyle changes.

Inhibitors. A high level of potassium (hyperkalemia) is a known side effect of Ace Inhibitors.

Beta Blockers. Normally, in cases of uncomplicated hypertension, the physician would perhaps select diuretics or beta blockers as the first line of choice for blood pressure treatment. However, because these drugs may cause high lipid levels and upset the control of diabetes mellitus, these are not the preferred treatment of choice for hypertension patients with diabetes mellitus. Beta blockers may also mask the effects of low blood sugar (hypoglycemia) and are therefore not considered to be the best agents for diabetics with hypertension.

Diuretics. Are diuretics completely safe to use when both diabetes and hypertension are present? Appropriate control of high blood pressure in diabetic patients is very important. In fact, as discussed earlier, the goal in the diabetics is to keep the blood pressure below 130/85 mmHg. Because of their side effect profile including a rise in blood sugar, diuretics are not considered to be the preferred class of medications for blood pressure in diabetics. Furthermore, the adverse effects of diuretics on cholesterol levels also increases the risk of developing heart disease.

Calcium Channel Blockers. Although calcium channel blockers are also considered a suitable choice for diabetic patients with hypertension, ACE Inhibitors are preferred. In one recent study published in *The New England Journal of Medicine* in 1998, Dr Estacio and his colleagues reported that although blood pressure control was adequate with both drugs, the ACE Inhibitors were definitely more useful in preventing deaths due to heart attacks. Based on these results, the authors considered the use of ACE inhibitors as superior.

It is obvious that with a wide variety of drugs available to control hypertension, there is little problem in bringing blood pressure under control with Ace Inhibitors alone or with combination therapy using beta blockers, calcium channel blockers or diuretics.

Hypertension and Insulin Resistance Syndrome (IRS)

It is important to understand a comparatively new term called 'insulin resistance syndrome' (IRS). Insulin resistance syndrome is characterised by a defect in the ability of insulin to push glucose into the muscles. In a normal person, when the blood sugar goes up, insulin is secreted from the pancreas. This insulin is necessary to push the glucose into the muscles and that keeps the blood sugar from going very high. However, in people with IRS, even though the insulin level is high, the insulin is unable to keep the blood sugar in normal range. In many ways, IRS is a pre-diabetic type of situation. The condition is most commonly seen in obese people. Typically, IRS has the following features:

- Obesity (mostly central obesity with excessive fat around the abdominal area).
- Lipid abnormalities (high triglyceride and low HDL).
- High level of blood insulin with high blood sugar.
- Hypertension.

Scientists and physicians have been interested in looking at the link between IRS and hypertension for more than two decades. Although no single cause has yet been determined, high levels of circulating insulin has been thought to cause hypertension.

Preventing IRS. Although genetic predisposition has been considered to contribute to the development of IRS, one can avoid IRS by simply avoiding obesity. Most people start gaining weight in their late 20s and continue to gain between 1.5 to 2 kgs each year. In other words, by the middle years, at the age of 45, a weight gain of about 20 kgs may have taken place. Dietary changes, restriction of salt and calories and regular aerobic exercise are important components of maintaining a healthy body weight.

Although research is likely to shed more light to the problem of IRS, because of the associated problem of obesity, hypertension, hyperlipidemia, diabetes mellitus and eventually coronary heart disease, this syndrome can prove to be a deadly one. People with poor dietary habits and a lazy lifestyle are particularly at risk of developing IRS. If you think you are one of those individuals, the time to act is now.

The following steps can help you in dealing with this problem.

1. Maintain ideal body weight. Do not accept weight gain as an inevitable part of advancing age.
2. Avoid high fat/high calorie food.
3. Maintain an active lifestyle with regular physical exercise.

4. Have fasting blood glucose checked every 6 to 12 months. Glucose intolerance* is an early indicator of risk of developing diabetes mellitus.
5. Have blood lipids checked at least once a year. People with insulin resistance syndrome often have high total cholesterol, triglyceride levels and low HDL levels.
6. Have blood pressure checked every 6 to 12 months. If your blood pressure is slowly creeping up along with weight gain, high fasting blood sugar, and lipid abnormalities, then you are perhaps close to joining the group of people suffering from insulin resistance syndrome.

References

1. Tight blood pressure control and risk of macrovascular and microvascular complications in type 2 diabetes: UKPDS 38. UK Prospective Diabetes Study Group. BMJ. 1998;317:703-713.
2. Weinsaft J W, O Rourke M F, Nichols W W, Sharma A M, Pischon T, Engeli S, Gavras H, Yusuf S, Francis G. Effect of Ramipril on Cardiovascular Events in High Risk Patients. N Engl J Med 2000; 343:64-66, Jul 6, 2000.

---

*Glucose Tolerance Levels

Normal	70 — 110mg
Glucose Intolerance	111 — 125mg
Diabetes	> 126mg

21

Hypertension and High Cholesterol

Men who love wisdom should acquaint themselves with a great many particulars.

Heraclitus

Hypertension is recognised as one of the three major risk factors for coronary heart disease. The other two major risk factors are smoking and high cholesterol. It is estimated that between 25 to 40 per cent of patients with hypertension also have high levels of blood cholesterol. The combination of high blood pressure and high cholesterol significantly increases the risk of death due to heart disease. In a landmark study (Multiple Risk Factor Intervention Trial[1]) 361,662 middle-aged men who were free of pre-existing coronary heart disease were studied over a 12 year period. Those with high blood pressure and high cholesterol were noted to have a much higher rate of death due to heart disease.

In a German study published in 1988, in *The American Heart Journal*, researchers found that, although high cholesterol is a more significant risk factor for coronary heart disease than hypertension or diabetes mellitus, the combination of these conditions was very dreadful.

In a paper published in *Cardiology in Review,* the world renowned physician, Dr William P. Castelli, Director of the Framingham Heart Study, called the combination of hypertension and high blood lipids as very dangerous and urged physicians to evaluate all hypertension patients for high lipid levels.

Lifestyle Changes

Undoubtedly, for someone with hypertension and noted to have high cholesterol, the risk of heart attack is more than additive. Therefore, it is very important to focus attention and control both hypertension as well as high cholesterol. The US Joint National Committee on Hypertension has strongly advised all physicians that hypertensive patients with high lipid levels must receive aggressive treatment for both conditions. Since lifestyle changes are likely to benefit both hypertension and high cholesterol, it is essential to change lifestyle.

Dietary Changes

Control of obesity requires dietary changes and regular physical exercise. Dietary changes including a reduction in the intake of saturated fat and cholesterol should help to bring cholesterol down. Salt intake must be kept to a minimum (see chapter 14).

Too much Alcohol is Dangerous

High alcohol consumption often leads to increased calorie intake and obesity. Therefore, daily alcohol intake should not be more than 1to 2 drinks per day. It would also be advisable to totally avoid alcohol for 2 to 3 days per week. All forms of alcohol including beer, wine and whisky contain calories. Most people end up eating a lot of extra calories in the form of snacks with alcohol.

Benefits of Physical Exercise

The need for physical exercise, especially of aerobic type, not only helps in weight loss but also controlling cholesterol and hypertension. No person is too old to start a regular physical exercise programme. In a recently published study in *Journal of American Geriatrics Society*, Dr Richard Pratley reported the effect of moderate intensity aerobic exercise in 17 elderly men over a period of nine months. It was found they were able to successfully lose weight with a significant reduction in their central obesity (fat around the abdomen). The patients were noted to have both lower cholesterol as well as lower blood pressure readings.

To Lower your Cholesterol

- Avoid being overweight. If possible keep body weight at least 5-7 kgs lighter than the ideal body weight.
- Limit alcohol intake to 1-2 drinks per day.
- Reduce salt intake to the minimum. Avoid table salt.
- Limit total fat intake to less than 30 per cent of total calories.
- Limit saturated fat intake to less than 10 per cent of total calories.
- Limit cholesterol intake to less than 300 mg per day.
- Increase intake of fibre, fruits and vegetables.

Adverse Effects of some Medications

Common medications used for the control of hypertension may also have some adverse metabolic effects including changes in blood sugar and lipid levels. Their effect on cholesterol, LDL, HDL and triglyceride levels is as below.

Effects of Anti-Hypertensive Medications on Lipids

Drugs	*Total Chol.*	*LDL*	*HDL*	*Triglyceride*
Diuretics	↑	↑	↓	↑
Beta blockers	↑	↑	↓	↑
ACE Inhibitors	—	—	—	—
Calcium channel blockers	—	—	—	—
Alpha blockers	↓	—	↑	—
Alpha & Beta blockers	—	—	—	—

— No effect, ↑ Increase, ↓ Decrease

The choice of appropriate medication has to be carefully weighed by the doctor. The doctor will also review other non-lipid side effects before choosing the best drug for treatment. Since some of the commonly used diuretics and beta blockers may raise total and LDL cholesterol by 10 to 20 per cent, the appropriate choice of medication becomes important. Drugs like Ace Inhibitors and calcium channel blockers have little effect on lipid levels and therefore may provide a better choice in the presence of high cholesterol.

References

1. The Multiple Risk Factor Intervention Trial. A National Study of Primary Prevention Coronary Heart Disease.*JAMA* 1976 Feb 23;235 (8):825-827.

22

Hypertension in Children

The joys of parents are secret, and so are their griefs and fears.

Francis Bacon

Although most discussion regarding high blood pressure is focussed on adults, it is important to understand that children and adolescents not immune to the problem of high blood pressure. In most families, parents simply do not think about such a possibility. It might be argued that if the parents could just take care of their own diseases, that would be just fine. However, children are the future wealth of any nation. In many cases, school health programmes perform a physical examination and, if during that examination, the blood pressure is found to be elevated, the parents of the child are informed by the school authorities.

Let us look at some of the issues involved with children and hypertension.

It is important to understand that the blood pressure of children varies with age, sex and even height. Blood pressure is considered to be high if the readings are higher than the 95th percentile for that group. The paediatrician, the child expert, is the one to know the normal and the abnormal levels of blood pressure for the child of any given age. For American children, the following normal blood pressure levels are recommended:

Normal Blood Pressure in Children

Age/yrs	*Boys*	*Girls*
1	104/58	105/59
6	115/75	112/73
12	125/82	124/81
17	138/88	130/85

Joint National Common Detection, Evaluation and Treatment

You would note that as children grow older, their normal values tend to be higher. It has been noted that if one or both parents have a history of hypertension, their children have a much higher risk of becoming hypertensive. Although, in most cases, this form of hereditary hypertension appears in the 30s or the 40s, the children may occasionally be found to develop hypertension in the early years.

If one or both parents suffer from hypertension, it is not really be a bad idea to take children for a regular routine check-up of blood pressure. In the words of Dr Claude Lenfant, the Director of US the National Heart, Lung and Blood Institute, 'Accurate blood pressure screening as a part of routine childhood examination is essential to both the current and future health of the nation's youth.'

Causes of Hypertension in Children. If a child's blood pressure is noted to be high, the doctor has to evaluate the underlying cause of hypertension. Is it the kidneys or adrenal glands or some other disease that is responsible for high blood pressure in a child of this age? Relevant laboratory and radiological tests may be necessary to help establish the diagnosis and/or to exclude the causes of secondary hypertension. If a treatable cause of hypertension is detected, the child can be expected to be spared from taking tablets for hypertension over the next 50 to 60 years of his life.

In many countries, hospitals and medical centres have specialised paediatrics hypertension clinics. In the absence of such specialised centres, it may be prudent to seek the expert opinion of an experienced paediatrician.

Most children with high blood pressure tend to be overweight. The need for regular exercise, diet control and weight loss cannot be over-emphasised. One of the major problems that both parents and physicians face is the problem of compliance. Can we expect the child to fully understand and adhere to the dietary and life-style changes? In such a situation, the type of food at home needs careful discussion with all family members. High fat and high salt food at home, would need to be substituted with low fat, low salt diet. Without this change the child is simply not going to be benefitted. In many ways, it is the whole family that may have to change its lifestyle. The child should be encouraged to maintain an active lifestyle and participate in the daily athletic activities. This is of course, helpful for weight loss and the general well-being of the child.

Medication. The choice of medications for children with hypertension is almost similar to that of adults. However, the doses have to be smaller and adjusted according to the blood pressure response. Fortunately, with appropriate lifestyle changes and medication use, the blood pressure can be safely controlled in all children and adolescents. Hypertension must never be ignored at any age, especially in children. In the absence of good control, high blood pressure can result in serious and life threatening complications and even premature death.

23

Old Age and High Blood Pressure

A medical revolution has extended the life of our older citizens without providing the dignity and security those later years deserve.

John F. Kennedy
1960

Blood pressure tends to rise with age. Generally speaking the term elderly (or senior citizens) is reserved for people aged 65 years and above. Several scientific studies have clearly shown a trend towards rising blood pressure with ageing.

There are at least five questions that must be answered regarding blood pressure and old age.

1. What happens to blood pressure with age?

2. How important is blood pressure control in old age?

3. Can blood pressure be safely treated in old age?

4. Is there a single best drug for treatment of hypertension in old age?

5. What if someone does not bother to take blood pressure medication in old age?

In the famous Framingham Heart Study, the blood pressure of 5209 men and women was monitored biannually for a period of thirty years and following observations noted.

- A rise of 20 mmHg in systolic and 10 mmHg in diastolic blood pressure between the ages of 30 and 60 years.
- In men, the blood pressure was noted to rise even in their 70s.
- In women systolic blood pressure continued to go up in their 80s as well.
- Over 65 per cent of adults were, thus, noted to develop hypertension over a thirty-year-period of observation.

In the US National Health and Nutrition Exam Survey, conducted between 1988 and 1991, it was noted that while hypertension affected only 4% of adults between the ages of 18 and 29, it affected 65% of adults over the age of 80. Hypertension, no doubt, is considered to be one of the commonest age-prevalent problems.

Both systolic as well as diastolic blood pressure start rising from the age of 20 onwards. While the systolic blood pressure continues to rise even after the age of 65, the diastolic blood pressure stops going up in old age.

Why should the blood pressure rise as one grows older? This question has been a matter of great research for many years. The hardening and narrowing of the arteries (arteriosclerosis) is considered to be the chief cause of the rise in blood pressure in old age.

Currently, all adults, irrespective of the age, are considered to have normal blood pressure only if their readings are below 140/90 mmHg. The new guidelines issued by the US Joint National Committee on Hypertension recommends that even in old age blood pressure must not be considered normal if it rises above 140/90 mmHg.

Treating Hypertension in the Elderly

Before the actual treatment for hypertension in old age is discussed, let us remember that:

1. Elderly people are usually less comfortable facing doctors or visiting big hospitals. The so-called 'white coat hypertension' phenomenon is far more common in older people.

2. Pseudohypertension, the condition of falsely elevated blood pressure, is a unique problem in older people. Before starting on any treatment the condition of pseudohypertension must be ruled out.

3. Just as in adults, in more than 95 per cent of older people the hypertension is of a primary (essential) type.

4. Postural hypotension is a common problem in the older persons. The blood pressure must be checked both in sitting as well standing positions to rule out the possibility of postural hypotension. Medication may also add to the problem of postural hypotension and cause

> It is estimated that in old age if you are able to lower your systolic blood pressure by 10 and diastolic by 5 mmHg you can cut down your risk of heart disease by 10 to 20 per cent.

dizziness, syncope and falls. It is therefore important to closely monitor the blood pressure and the side effects of treatment in older people.

Investigations in the Elderly Require

Let the doctor decide what tests are important. In most cases you do not need an exhaustive battery of tests. Simple blood tests, urine tests, chest X-ray and electrocardiography (ECG) are generally sufficient for assessment. Treatment of hypertension in old age is certainly beneficial in reducing the long-term complications of hypertension. The general principles of management of high blood pressure are not very different in old age. Lifestyle changes are helpful for all adults, including the elderly. These include dietary control; weight reduction; salt reduction; stop smoking; and regular exercise.

Making Lifestyle Changes

Do the lifestyle changes work in older people? Many patients in their 60s and 70s have often asked this question. Not only that, but even some physicians seem not to attach much significance to lifestyle changes in reducing blood pressure in old age.

In a recent trial of nonpharmacological approach of blood pressure treatment in the elderly, Dr Whelton and his colleagues[1] studied a group of 975 obese and non obese patients, 60 to 80 years old, who had their blood pressure controlled with a single antihypertensive medication. Those who were taking lower amounts of salt (1800mg or less) and were able to lose weight (4.5kg or more) were noted to require at least 30 per cent lower doses of the same medication to keep their blood pressure under control. These scientists therefore concluded that older patients must always be advised to lower their body weight and salt intake in order to control their hypertension.

Before any medication is started, it is important to understand that there are increased chances of complications of drug treatment in old age. In general, medications cause more side effects in the elderly. While on the one hand the control of hypertension in the elderly is as important as in younger adults, drugs do tend to cause more problems in later years of life due to altered drug absorption, altered liver and kidney function, decreased baroreceptor activity and greater likelihood of drug to drug interaction because of use of multiple medication.

Benefits of Treatment in the Elderly

There is a broad consensus of medical opinion that high blood pressure in old age must be treated. Dr Madhavan and his colleagues[2] in their study found that older patients with high systolic blood pressure and normal or even lower diastolic blood pressure had a much higher risk of heart attacks. Isolated systolic hypertension (ISH) is a condition that is mainly seen in older people. This condition is characterised by presence of high (over 140 mmHg) systolic blood pressure, while the diastolic blood pressure is usually normal. Until recently, physicians did not consider ISH as a significant medical problem. However, we now know better. ISH is not considered a part of normal ageing process and therefore ISH does need proper treatment for control of blood pressure.

High Blood Pressure in Old Age: 7 Golden Rules

1 Blood pressure control (less than 140/90) is essential for all adults, including the elderly.

2 Since blood pressure tends to rise with ageing, there is a need to have blood pressure checked at least twice a year by a doctor.

3 The main choice of medications is between diuretics, beta receptor blockers, calcium channel blockers, and ACE Inhibitors. Let the doctor decide which is the best drug combination.

4 Almost always start with a small dose. With monitoring, the doses can be adjusted accordingly.

5 Be familiar with the side effects of all medications. If you suspect that you may be having one or more side effects, consult your physician. Do not stop taking the medication. Some of the medications, such as beta receptor blockers, if stopped abruptly, may lead to rebound hypertension.

6 Once the blood pressure is adequately controlled, the frequency of visits to the physician can be reduced. However, it is advisable that the physician be visited at least every 3 to 6 months.

7 Always remind yourself about the importance of a strict control. It is only through good control that you can reduce the risk of serious complications such as stroke, heart attack and kidney failure.

The World Health Organization (WHO) in its most recent guidelines agreed that systolic readings of over 140 (with diastolic less than 90) should be considered as isolated systolic hypertension (ISH) and all patients with ISH need to consult their physicians for blood pressure control.

The dangers of ignoring the control of hypertension in old age have become very clear. In a study published in *The Lancet*, in 1997, Dr Staessen and his colleagues demonstrated a significant reduction in the incidence of heart attacks and heart failure in older patients treated for their hypertension. More recently, in 1997, Dr Kostis and his colleagues similarly published the positive benefits of controlling hypertension in old age in *The Journal of American Medical Association.*

In the Systolic Hypertension in Europe (Syst-Eur) trial, patients 60 years and older were noted to benefit with active treatment of hypertension. There was a 26 per cent reduction in cardiovascular events in non diabetic patients and 69 per cent reduction in the diabetic group, along with a significant decline in fatal and non fatal strokes (38 per cent in non diabetics and 73 per cent in diabetic patients). Beneficial results have also been reported from systolic hypertension in a Chinese study (Syst-China) confirming that active and aggressive treatment of hypertension in old age can protect you from stroke and heart disease, the two most dreadful complications of hypertension.

Similarly, with the reduction of blood pressure, the risk of left ventricular hypertrophy and congestive heart failure can be reduced significantly. Unfortunately, too many older people ignore the value of their blood pressure control.

References

1. V L Burt, P Whelton, E J Roccella, et al., 'Prevalence of Hypertension in the US Adult Population: Results from the Third National Health and Nutrition Examination Survey, 1988-1991', Hypertension 25 (3) (1995), pp. 303-304.
2. Madhavan S Ooi W L Cohen H, Alderman M H: Relation of pulse pressure reduction to the incidence of myocardial infarction. Hypertension 1994: 395 401.

24

Quality of Life and Treatment of Hypertension

Look to your health, and if you have it praise God and value it next to a good conscience; for, health is the second blessing that we mortals are capable of: a blessing that money can not buy, and therefore value it and be thankful for it.

Izaak Walton
1676

It is difficult to define what exactly is QOL. QOL may mean different things to different people. Although no satisfactory definition is as yet available, the following components have been considered to be important in the determination of QOL:

- Sense of life satisfaction including cheerfulness, happiness, absence of fatigue, anxiety and depression.

- Intellectual functioning (ability to concentrate, alertness, and memory).
- Social functioning (ability to interact with family, friends and colleagues).
- Emotional well-being.
- Physical well-being (tiredness, lethargy, headache, loss of taste, dizziness and sexual functioning).

In the 1980's scientists started to look into the impact of medications on the Quality Of Life (QOL) of those on medicines to control hypertension. The question of QOL becomes particularly important since in most cases, patients with mild or moderate hypertension hardly have any symptoms. If these patients can be persuaded to take medication for the control of hypertension, they are unlikely to suffer from symptoms arising from the side effects of drugs used for lowering blood pressure once it becomes higher. Additionally, it has become clear that if QOL is impaired, they are not likely to take the treatment for the rest of their lives.

Physicians and scientists often talk about the problem of noncompliance with medications. I personally have known several patients who had serious side effects with medications commonly used in the late 1960s and early 1970s. No wonder many of these patients simply stopped taking medication because of persistent side effects interfering with their QOL. I am sure most physicians can tell you similar stories about medication use and side effects.

The 'Quality Of Life' Concept. The whole concept of QOL is somewhat new in the field of medical practice. The need to address the question of QOL was realised mainly because of the following reasons:

1. If a disease like hypertension is largely asymptomatic, i.e., causing no symptoms, why would any patient tolerate symptoms caused by drug treatment?

2. Non compliance continues to be a major problem in the treatment of hypertension. It is estimated that between 25 to 40 per cent of hypertensive patients do not take medications as directed.

3. If the QOL of a patient is likely to be impaired with the treatment, the patient is likely to be reluctant to continue the treatment.

Do newer antihypertensive drugs offer better efficacy and quality of life with fewer side effects? Recent scientific studies have tried to answer these questions.

In the treatment of hypertension, physicians are often too much focussed on simply reducing the blood pressure. In one interesting study, Dr Jachuck and his colleagues[1] reviewed a total of 74 hypertensive patients. They questioned the patients, their spouses and doctors regarding the QOL of these patients. While almost all physicians reported that the patients' QOL had improved, only 50 per cent of the patients agreed with their doctors' assessment. Almost half of these patients felt that their overall QOL was worse with the treatment.

How do we explain the difference in this perception? The answer is clear. The physicians are only looking at the blood pressure numbers and not giving enough attention to the overall QOL.

In any discussion of QOL, therefore, several factors need to be considered carefully:

- Is the blood pressure properly controlled?
- How often is the medication taken during the day? Taking medication only once a day is considered to be associated with better QOL.
- Are there any side effects?
- How serious are the side effects? If the intake of a blood pressure pill has caused significant emotional, physical or sexual disturbance, QOL cannot be considered to be good. If a drug is causing a feeling of tiredness and lethargy and the individual to be so tired and lethargic that he/she does not even feel like going to work then he/she is not likely to continue taking the medication.

In one of the major research studies of QOL, Dr Croog and his colleagues[2] compared the three major classes of drugs including ACE Inhibitors (Captopril), Methyl-dopa (Aldomet), and beta blocker (Propranolol). While only 7 per cent of patients on ACE Inhibitors had to stop taking medications because of adverse drug reactions, 12 per cent of patients on beta blockers and as many as 20 per cent on Aldomet had to stop taking their medications because of associated side effects.

So it becomes very important for everyone to be aware of the issue of QOL and discuss any side effects or problems associated with the treatment being prescribed by the doctor. Although it is very important to make yourself familiar with the side effects of the medications, it is not always easy to figure out whether any new symptoms being experienced are a part of the disease, i.e.

Medication: Once, Twice, or Thrice a Day?

Like millions of other patients, I am sure you would prefer to take the medication only once a day instead of twice or three times a day. Many studies have also concluded that if a medication is to be taken 2-4 times a day, the chances of compliance are diminished proportionately.

Let us say you were prescribed a beta-blocker for twice a day to be taken at 9 am and 9 pm. If you took only the 9 am dose, it may result in poor control of blood pressure towards the late evening hours. Because stroke and heart attacks are far more common in the early morning hours, if you missed the 9 pm dose, your blood pressure may not be fully controlled in the early morning hours and, therefore, you are putting yourself at risk simply because you missed the 9 pm dose as advised.

In recent years, some drug companies have even tried to develop skin patches (clonidine, for example) that may need to be changed only once or twice a week.

It is important to note that the goal is to keep blood pressure under control for the period of 24 hours in the day.

hypertension, or is it caused by the treatment? Only a thorough discussion with the physician can help to understand these issues.

It is obviously difficult to accept any treatment that is worse than the disease itself. Fortunately, with better research and understanding of the problems associated with earlier antihypertensive medications like reserpine or methyl-dopa, we now have much better groups of drugs. While physicians are commonly using these drugs to control hypertension, it is you — the patient — who needs to become an active partner in the management of your hypertension. Remember, the more you know about your disease and your treatment choices, the better it is for your long-term health and happiness. Hypertension is no longer considered to be a matter of purely controlling the blood pressure numbers. It is very important that you enjoy a good quality of life with good control of blood pressure. Fortunately, it is possible to achieve those two goals at the same time.

References

1. Jachuck S J, Bierley H, Jachuck S, Willcox P M. The effect of hypotensive drugs on the quality of life. J Roy Coll Gen Pract 1982;32:103-5.
2. Williams G H, Croog S H, Levine S, Testa M A, Sudilovsky A. Impact of antihypertensive therapy on quality of life: effect of hydrochlorothiazide. J Hypertens Suppl. 1987 Feb;5(1):S29-35.

25

Hypertension and Hormonal Treatment

Of all the ailments which may blow out life's little candle, heart disease is the chief.

William Boyd

Post-menopausal years refer to the years of life after women stop menstruating, generally between the age of 45 to 55 years. Because hormonal levels of estrogen drop after this age, women commonly tend to have an increased risk of heart disease as well as osteoporosis (thinning of the bones).

If you are taking hormones like estrogens or corticosteroids for any reason, the blood pressure may increase. Estrogen intake has been on the rise in recent years particularly because of greater awareness of the fact that hormonal replacement is associated with reduced risk of osteoporosis and heart disease in post-menopausal years.

Hypertension after Menopause. Women in general, tend to develop more hypertension after menopause. Although no precise explanation is available, it has been suggested that, before menopause, because of the monthly menstruation, there is a reduction of fluid volume. Messerli and his colleagues[1] in 1987 suggested that before menopause, women have a higher cardiac output and heart rate and lower peripheral vascular resistance, all probably due to a higher amount of circulating estrogens. Whatever the underlying cause for hypertension in post-menopausal years, the overall risk of cardiovascular complications does go up in women after the age of 50 years.

Pros and Cons of Hormonal Replacement Therapy. In general, for many years it has been believed that hormonal replacement therapy does not increase the risk of hypertension and, in fact, because of a beneficial effect of high HDL level, provides an overall protection to the heart.

With hormonal treatment, there are definite benefits in the symptoms of menopause including reduction of hot flashes and night sweats and strengthening of bones (prevention of osteoporosis). In the Western world, between 20 to 40 per cent of women are estimated to take hormonal replacement treatment during menopause. Recent studies have, however, questioned the cardiovascular benefits of hormonal replacement therapy.

While the issue of long-term cardiovascular benefits or risks of hormonal treatment still remains unclear, it is important to have blood pressure checked regularly (at least every 3 to 6 months) for any woman if currently taking hormonal replacement therapy (estrogen or estrogen and progesterone together). If the blood pressure is noted to be going up, the physician may advise stopping the hormones altogether. Alternatively, if the hormone treatment is considered to be absolutely essential, some additional medications to control hypertension may also be advised.

As a word of caution, hormonal replacement therapy also raises the risk of breast and uterine cancer. Therefore, the need for a regular check up from your gynaecologist cannot be under-emphasised.

References

1. Messerli F H, Baravaglia G E, Schmieder R E, Sundaard R E, Sundaard -Riise K, Nunez B D, Amodeo C 1987 Disparate cardiovascular findings in men and women with essential hypertension. Ann Intern Med. 107:158-161.

26

Hypertension in Pregnancy

Childhood is the kingdom where no one dies.

Edna St. Vincent

During pregnancy, the body experiences significant changes in blood volume, cardiac output, peripheral vascular resistance, kidney and uterine blood flow. At least ten different hormonal changes have an impact on blood pressure. In normal pregnancy, blood pressure usually goes down in the first two trimesters. During the last or third trimester, the blood pressure returns to normal levels. Because of the fact that blood pressure usually falls in the first six months of pregnancy, women with a previous history of hypertension may have normal blood pressure readings.

Hypertension occurs in 5-10 per cent of all pregnancies. Many women (approximately 4 to 17 per cent) who have had hypertension during their pregnancies will continue to have high blood pressure after delivery. If the pregnancy is complicated with hypertension, the baby may have a low birth weight. However, hypertension is not a contraindication to becoming pregnant.

Pre-Eclampsia and Eclampsia. What is pre-eclampsia? If a pregnant woman develops high blood pressure after 20 weeks of pregnancy and has significant loss of protein in the urine (proteinuria) as well as excessive swelling (oedema) of the legs, the pregnancy is said to be complicated with pre-eclampsia.

Pre-eclampsia is typically a disease of the first pregnancy, but if someone has had pre-eclampsia in the first pregnancy, the risk of developing pre-eclampsia in the second and subsequent pregnancies is much higher than a woman who had no such problems during her first pregnancy. Women with twins, diabetes mellitus, kidney disease or a family history of pre-eclampsia are also noted to have a high risk of pre-eclampsia.

All women with suspected pre-eclampsia need very close medical supervision preferably in a hospital setting, where an experienced physician can control the hypertension and monitor blood tests. Delivery is best induced at or near the term. Women with severe hypertension may also need to have induced delivery but such decisions are best left to the obstetrician.

In eclampsia, the woman develops seizures (fits) in addition to hypertension, proteinuria and oedema.

Hypertension increases the risk of pre-eclampsia and eclampsia during pregnancy. Although simple hypertension alone may be less of a problem in pregnancy, these conditions are far more serious and can even prove to be life-threatening.

While the specific treatment of pre-eclampsia and eclampsia is beyond the scope of this book, it is sufficient to understand that all stages of hypertension in pregnancy require immediate treatment and close observation.

Monitoring the health of Mother and Foetus. The health of the mother as well as of the unborn child requires attention in the treatment of hypertension in pregnancy. To achieve the best results, the treatment decisions should be taken both by the physician as well as the obstetrician. The doctors must not only keep the goal of preventing complications in the mother alone, but also ensure that the unborn baby is not harmed by the treatment for hypertension.

Gradual reduction of blood pressure is important to avoid a sudden drop in the placental blood flow and harm to the foetus.

Finally, close and careful monitoring of blood pressure during pregnancy is important in all cases. If there is any suspicion of high blood pressure, it may not be a bad idea to buy a home blood pressure machine and record your blood pressure at least once a day. If the readings remain abnormally high, you must visit your doctor far more frequently.

27

Hypertension in Athletes

Good health is a serious business. Like life itself, it has to be worked at and it takes on added meaning with effort.

Norman Cousins
1989

It is widely known that a physically fit individual is less likely to develop a disease like hypertension. However, being physical fit and interested in athletic activities do not provide absolute immunity against hypertension. Athletes with a family history of hypertension, for example, are still at considerable risk of developing hypertension. Fortunately, with better understanding of the disease and the availability of several types of medications, it has become possible to continue with daily physical exercise and sports.

There are, however, a few important issues to be remembered.

If found to be hypertensive, the devastating effects of untreated hypertension must not be ignored even though you feel fit and enjoy a lot of stamina at the current time. Just like any other person who is not an athlete, there are likely to be the same complications of hypertension if blood pressure remains uncontrolled for several years. Under all circumstances, it is important to seek appropriate medical help and get blood pressure under control.

Try to get involved in the isotonic (aerobic) type of exercise. It has been noted that the aerobic exercises are by far more helpful in the control and reduction of blood pressure than after exercises. Brisk walking, jogging, running, cycling and swimming, are all aerobic exercises. In general, isometric exercises such as weight lifting, are noted to be associated with a rise in blood pressure.

Selection of the right medications for hypertension in individuals with an athletic lifestyle has received a lot of attention. While beta blockers and diuretics have been recommended as the first choice for uncomplicated hypertension, these drugs may interfere with performance for those involved in competitive sports.

28

Hypertensive Emergency Care

He is the best physician that knows the worthlessness of most medicines.

Benjamin Franklin
1733

If blood pressure is notoriously elevated to a very high level, there is likely to be a need for urgent treatment. In most cases, the blood pressure shoots up to high levels only in hypertension cases which have remained ignored and untreated for a long time. If the blood pressure is not brought down to satisfactory levels, there is risk of brain haemorrhage and even a rupture of the aorta. Brain and eye damage, kidney failure and stroke are other major consequences of persistently high blood pressure.

In many cases of dangerously elevated blood pressure, the blood pressure of patients requiring emergency treatment is found to be between 200 and 220 mmHg systolic and 115 and 130 mmHg of diastolic readings.

In recent years, the percentage of people getting into a state of hypertensive crisis has gone down substantially.

The conditions which are often associated with excessively high blood pressure readings may require urgent treatment.

Patients with hypertensive emergencies often require hospital admission for careful observation and monitoring of their blood pressure. They need a thorough examination to look into the possible cause of the sudden rise in blood pressure. In addition, they routinely require full assessment, with blood tests (electrolytes, glucose, BUN, urea, creatinine) ECG and chest x-ray, etc. If not performed previously, the doctor may also order specialised tests to rule out the secondary causes of hypertension including renovascular hypertension and pheochromocytoma (a tumour of the adrenal gland), etc.

In a situation of hypertensive emergency, the blood pressure needs to be reduced substantially within a period of one to two hours. To quickly bring down the blood pressure, medications are commonly administered by injection.

A detailed description and evaluation of the medications used for hypertensive emergencies may be beyond the scope of this book. In almost all cases, the decision to select the right medication has to be made by the doctor after careful evaluation. However, a brief discussion of the commonly used drugs for urgent reduction of blood pressure is in order.

Nitroprusside. Sodium nitroprusside, given intravenously, has an immediate effect in lowering the blood pressure. Acting directly on the walls of the blood vessels, nitroprusside dilates the arterial as well as the venous system. However, if nitroprusside is used for more than 2 to 3 days, patients may experience thiocyanate toxicity (blurred vision, sensation of pins and needles and mental confusion). Your doctor will especially need to monitor liver and kidney functions as well with the use of nitroprusside.

Nitroglycerin. As compared to nitroprusside, nitroglycerin is somewhat safer even for patients with heart disease and compromised liver and kidney functions. Nitroglycerin is a vasodilator and may cause headaches, nausea and slow heart rate as side effects.

Labetalol. Labetalol is a beta blocker and is especially useful for patients with high blood pressure resulting from pheochromocytoma, cocaine toxicity or following coronary artery bypass surgery. Once the blood pressure is controlled, labetalol can also be given orally.

Esmolol. Esmolol is a short acting beta blocker. If the patient also has significant heart failure, esmolol may worsen the heart failure. Esmolol is considered to be helpful if the high levels of blood pressure are associated with aortic dissection, a tear in the innermost layer of the aorta.

Nicardipine. Nicardipine is a calcium channel blocker. Excessive fall of blood pressure, headache and rapid heart rate are some of the side effects.

Enalaprilat. Enalaprilat is an ACE Inhibitor type of medication. Given intravenously, it is quite effective in lowering the blood pressure. The drug may also be given with diuretics to enhance its blood pressure-lowering effects.

Nifedipine. Nifedipine, a calcium channel blocker, is a fast acting drug and, until recently, was widely used for rapid reduction of blood pressure. However, nifedipine can sometimes cause an excessive drop in the blood pressure and can lead to reflex tachycardia and uncontrolled rise in the heart rate. In some cases, patients have also been known to have heart attacks and sudden strokes with the use of nifedipine. Because of these reasons, oral nifedipine must never be used to treat the emergency hypertensive state.

If blood pressure is noted to be high (systolic between 170 and 200 mmHg and diastolic between 110 and 120), yet there does not seem to be a hypertensive crisis, the doctor may choose to treat with bigger doses of one or more oral medications. A variety of drugs including clonidine, diuretics, beta blockers and calcium channel blockers can serve this purpose.

29

Home Blood Pressure Monitoring

Healing is a matter of time, but it is sometimes also a matter of opportunity.

Hippocrates
460-375 BC

With the advancement of technology, small portable blood pressure machines have become widely available. Most of these handy machines cost between Rs. 2,000-5,000. There are several types and models of small blood pressure machines available in the market. The most common varieties are mercury or aneroid manometers. Over the years there has been a great improvement in these products and nowadays you can purchase blood pressure machines with cuffs that are easy to put around the arm. Almost all these machines have a push-button system for the inflation of the cuffs. Additionally, these modern machines have digital readouts and also a memory system that can record several recent readings. Some companies have also introduced finger or wrist blood pressure monitor machines. However, the accuracy of finger and wrist monitors is not considered to be great. Based on my own experience with these machines, I would suggest that you go in for a good quality arm- cuff type of model.

Two simple steps are important to understand before you can consider your home blood pressure machine to be reliable and helpful.

First, please read the accompanying instructions very carefully.

Second, you need to establish the accuracy of the machine. The simplest and the best way to do that is to take your own machine on the next visit to the doctor and have blood pressure checked with both the standard sphygmomanometer in the clinic as well as your own machine. If the readings from your machine are not very different from the readings taken by the clinic's sphygmomanometer, then you can consider your home machine to be reliable. At least once a year this exercise should be repeated so that there is assurance of consistency and accuracy of your home blood pressure machine.

How Efficient are the Blood Pressure Monitoring Machines?

Home blood pressure measurement has received its seal of approval as a result of many scientific studies. In most cases, it has been noted that home blood pressure readings are more accurate than readings taken in doctors, offices. The problem of anxiety and pressure-stress response in the doctor's office (white coat hypertension) has already been discussed. Studies have tried to correlate the home blood pressure readings with more sophisticated ambulatory blood pressure recording machines (small machines attached to the body). It has been noted that the home readings are much closer to the true blood pressure readings noted from the ambulatory blood pressure machines. The readings taken in doctors' offices have been found to be generally higher.

Dr Thomas G. Pickering, a world renowned hypertension expert from Cornell Medical Center in New York, strongly believes that home blood pressure monitoring can make a big difference in improving the quality of treatment of hypertension.

In recent years, the use of home blood pressure measurement has been on the rise. The sixth report of the US Joint National Committee strongly favoured home blood pressure monitoring. In its report, the Committee declared that 'measurement of blood pressure outside of the clinician's office may provide valuable information for the initial evaluation of patients with hypertension and for monitoring the response to treatment.' The World Health Organization has also emphasised the positive role of out of office blood pressure measurements.

Do Patients do a Good Job of Measuring their own Blood Pressure? In a study reported in the *American Journal of Hypertension*[1] several blood pressure readings taken by patients were compared to recordings from ambulatory instruments and readings taken by doctors in their offices. Interestingly, it was found that readings taken at home by patients themselves correlated well with ambulatory as well as office blood pressure readings.

There are several different areas where home measurement of blood pressure can be very helpful:

1. Home blood pressure measurements can be immensely helpful in establishing the diagnosis of hypertension, especially if blood pressure readings are

high-normal. If a visit to the doctor's office has made you aware of the fact that your blood pressure is in the high-normal range (close to 140/90), you need to know whether you really have hypertension. The best course in such circumstances is to make a small investment in health and buy a home blood pressure machine. Learning to use this apparatus is not difficult. Take 2 to 3 readings per day, at different times, each time after resting for a few minutes. Make a note of all the readings and next time you visit the doctor, go over these readings. A list of multiple home readings will help your doctor in establishing the diagnosis of hypertension.

2. Home blood pressure readings can also be helpful in evaluating the impact of lifestyle changes. If blood pressure is marginally high, and you are making your best efforts to change your lifestyle, you would certainly like to know whether your blood pressure has, in fact, gone down or not. Surely, a drop of 5 to 10 mmHg will convince you about the real value of lifestyle changes. Almost certainly you will feel encouraged and perhaps pursue those lifestyle changes more vigorously.

3. A personal record of multiple readings will help you to see if your blood pressure is in good control or not. Remember, your goal is to keep the blood pressure below 140/90 at all times. In some cases, if you already have some evidence of damage to your vital organs as a result of hypertension (kidney failure, coronary heart disease, or heart failure), your doctor may have to set a lower target for the control of your blood pressure. Multiple home blood pressure readings can prove to be immensely helpful in achieving the desirable blood pressure control.

4. If you are taking 3 to 4 pills for the control of your blood pressure, and if the home monitoring reveals that your blood pressure is much lower than what it used to be, it may be time to reduce your medication. Once again, multiple readings taken at home can help you to get a better picture of the overall control of hypertension and discuss the ongoing treatment choices and modifications with your doctor.

5. Home blood pressure monitoring can also help in ruling out the problem of white coat hypertension. If you are a nervous type of person, your blood pressure is more likely to shoot up when you visit a doctor. In such cases, home blood pressure monitoring can provide tremendous help in avoiding a false diagnosis. Why get yourself falsely labelled as hypertensive just because on a couple of visits to the doctor's office your blood pressure was noted to be high. If actual blood pressure readings taken at home are available, the physician may attribute this discrepancy to white coat hypertension.

Home blood pressure monitoring is being recognised as playing an important role in the detection and management of hypertension. In the words of Dr Norman Kaplan and Dr Raymond W. Gifford Jr., the two noted hypertension experts in the United States, 'Just like home glucose monitoring in diabetes mellitus, home blood pressure monitoring plays an important role in the management of hypertension'.

References

1. Brueren MM, Van Limpt P, Schouten HJA, et al. Is a series of blood pressure measurements by the general practitioner or the patient a reliable alternative to ambulatory blood pressure measurement? A study in general practice with reference to short-term and long-term between visit variability. *Am J Hypertens* (Aug) 1997; 10:879-885.

Risk Assessment for High Blood Pressure

Causes	*Likely*	*Not Likely*	
Heredity			
One parent has high blood pressure	☐	☑	
Both parents have high blood pressure	☑	☐	
Neither parent has high blood pressure	☐	☑	
Age			
Under 40 years	☐	☑	
Between 40-65 years	☑	☐	More likely in women.
Weight			
> 10-15% of optimum weight	☑	☐	See p. 141
Diet			
Largely processed fatty meats, preserved fish, dairy food & refined canned food, snacks	☑	☐	
High Salt Diet	☑	☐	

Causes	Likely	Not Likely	
Personality Types			
Type A Personality	☑	☐	
Type B Personality	☐	☑	See p. 127
Regular Smoking			
> 4 cigarettes a day	☑	☐	Nicotine acclerates heart rate.
Contraceptive Pill	☑	☐	Regular check-up advisable.
Alcohol			
Consumption of > 100 ml daily	☑	☐	

Glossary

Auscultation (by stethoscope): An aid to diagnose abnormalities of the heart, lungs, intestines and other organs based on the changes in sound patterns caused by different disease processes.

Baroreceptor: A collection of sensory nerve endings specialised to monitor changes in blood pressure.

Benign prostatic hypertrophy (BPH): This is not related with cancer of the prostate which is an entirely different disease.

Bronchospasm: Narrowing of bronchi by muscular contraction in response to some stimulus as in asthma and bronchitis.

Captopril tests: A special scan using an ace-inhibitor type of drug.

Cushing's syndrome: Condition resutling from excess amounts of corticosteroid hormones in the body. Symptoms include weight gain, reddening of the face and neck, raised blood pressure, and raised blood glucose levels.

Gynaecomastia: A condition characterised by painful enlargement of the breast.

Haemolytic anaemia: It is due to red-cell destruction.

Homeostasis: Physiological process by which the internal body systems (blood pressure, body temperature) are maintained at equilibrium, despite variations in the external condition.

Hypertensive Encephalopathy: Any of various diseases that affect the functioning of the brain.

Lupus like syndrome: Lupus is a connective tissue disease.

Palpation by fingers: Process of examining part of the body by careful feeling with the hands and fingertips.

Peripheral resistance: Constrictions and dilatation of the vessels.

Postural hypotension: A condition in which one feels dizzy or faint when standing up too quickly.

Spironolactone: A synthetic corticosteroid used to treat high blood pressure, heart failure and fluid retention.

Sympathetic nervous system: One of the two divisions of the antonomic nervous system, having fibres that leaves the central nervous system.

❑❑❑